CBT for Psychological Well-Being

T0258511

CBT for Psychological Well-Being in Cancer

A Skills Training Manual Integrating DBT, ACT, Behavioral Activation and Motivational Interviewing

Dr. Mark Carlson

WILEY Blackwell

Registered Offices
John Wiley & Sons, Inc., 111 River Street, Hoboken, NJ 07030, USA
John Wiley & Sons Ltd, The Atrium, Southern Gate, Chichester, West Sussex, PO19 8SQ, UK

Editorial Office
The Atrium, Southern Gate, Chichester, West Sussex, PO19 8SQ, UK

For details of our global editorial offices, customer services, and more information about Wiley products visit us at www.wiley.com.

Wiley also publishes its books in a variety of electronic formats and by print-on-demand. Some content that appears in standard print versions of this book may not be available in other formats.

Library of Congress Cataloging-in-Publication Data applied for.

ISBN 9781119161431

Cover image © kwasny221/Gettyimages

Set in 10/12.5pt GalliardStd by Aptara Inc., New Delhi, India

10 9 8 7 6 5 4 3 2 1

This work is dedicated to my son, Spencer.

Thank you for sharing the world through your experience: You stop to see the beauty when others rush by, you love without condition, you laugh with your whole being, you open your heart to all around you, you are strong in life, you have an undying curiosity, you find hope and compassion when many do not, you believe, and you are amazing! I hope that you stay connected to who you are and what you are capable of doing even in times of pain and diversity. Know that I love you with all of my being, I will always be with you, and I am proud to be your dad.

Contents

Acknowledgments

I would like to thank my team for making this work a reality.

Brittany Hamann – for all of your hard work, contributions, and dedication to this project.
Meagan Karsten – for your passion and contributions.
Dr. Amy Gimbel – for your willingness to do whatever is needed and for your contributions.
Dr. Morgan Cusack – for believing in this work and your dedication.
Dr. Lane Pederson – for your friendship and drive.
Shelley – for your support and stability.
Dr. Steve Girardeau – for your wisdom and guidance.
The entire team at Wiley.
Mom and Dad – for your unwavering support.
Julie – for being there every step of the way!

Chapter 1

Introduction to CBT for Psychological Well-Being in Cancer: Orientation to the Manual

When the word "cancer" is mentioned, people typically pay attention. When it is in the context of a medical appointment, or when discussing testing results, one of our biggest fears may become reality. Most everyone knows someone with cancer. There are stories of triumphs and stories of pain in every family. Reactions to the diagnosis of cancer, its treatment, and its course vary greatly between individuals. Although individual reactions may be quite different, there are many common themes found in what is experienced and what is needed. The first main theme is that cancer affects an individual's functioning and their quality of life. The other main themes can be organized into biological, psychological, and social perspectives. The focus of this manual is to address the complex needs of individuals diagnosed with cancer. Since there are more than 100 types of cancer, I have chosen not to focus on any one specific type. It seemed more appropriate to address the common reactions and issues that individuals with cancer experience. This is not designed to be an exhaustive and all-inclusive work, but rather another step in the direction toward treating the whole person.

Chapter 2 provides an overview of cancer statistics and treatments, to orient the reader to the enormity of the impact of cancer. Chapter 3 outlines a proposed treatment structure that addresses flexible treatment modalities for the professional. Chapter 4 makes up the bulk of the manual, and is organized into four sections: general, biological, psychological, and social. The general section consists of six headings that orient the clinician to the treatment of this population, ranging from skills training to work with safety issues. The biological section addresses themes such as treatment compliance and self-advocacy. The psychological section addresses issues of anxiety, depression, finding meaning, and more. The social section focuses on the individual's needs, as well as the needs of their support systems and strategies to increase healthy interactions.

Each section of Chapter 4 is presented with an outline of its contents, beginning with an introduction to the topic and points of discussion. The discussion points can

CBT for Psychological Well-Being in Cancer: A Skills Training Manual Integrating DBT, ACT, Behavioral Activation and Motivational Interviewing, First Edition. Mark Carlson.
© 2017 John Wiley & Sons, Ltd. Published 2017 by John Wiley & Sons, Ltd.

be covered in either group or individual therapy as a way to ground the individual and explore their experience. The sections then transition into sets of skills to teach, which are designed to increase the patient's functioning and quality of life. They also provide assessments tools, which can be used to track progress or identify key aspects of the patient's functioning. Participants are encouraged to practice the skill sets in session using handouts, and to generalize what they are learning outside of the therapeutic sessions by completing the homework assignments/tracking tools and reviewing them in the following session. The sections conclude with notes to the clinician, which are designed to highlight key points and provide suggestions.

There is no "right" way to incorporate a manualized approach. The goal is to focus on the needs of the individual seeking services, while striving to increase their functioning and quality of life. Our health care system is moving toward integrated health care. This manual is designed to assist in narrowing the gap between health care professions by integrating different treatment approaches in order to increase overall health and wellness. The World Health Organization (1948) defines health as a state of complete physical, mental, and social well-being, and not merely the absence of disease or infirmity. This definition has not changed since it was adopted in 1948, and I hope this work will help clinicians move in the direction of embracing it.

Chapter 2

Cancer Statistics and the Scope of the Topic

The prevalence and cost of cancer are a growing concern in the United States and beyond our borders. There is an immense need for coordination of medical and psychological management to treat individuals suffering with cancer and residual conditions that often result from the disease. The American Cancer Society reported that in 2013 "about 1,660,290 new cancer cases are expected to be diagnosed in the US", with "about 580,350 Americans…expected to die of cancer, almost 1,600 people per day." It further estimated that in 2014 there were 14.5 million Americans alive with a history of cancer and that by 2024 there will be 19 million. Currently in the United States, "men have a 1 in 2 lifetime risk of developing cancer; for women, the risk is a little more than 1 in 3" (American Cancer Society, 2013). "Cancer is the second most common cause of death in the US, exceeded only by heart disease, [accounting] for about 1 of every 4 deaths in 2013" (American Cancer Society, 2013). Nearly one-fourth of people with chronic conditions also reported experiencing limitations to daily activity due to their illness and experienced clinical mental health concerns. "The 5-year relative survival rate for all persons diagnosed with cancer between 2002 and 2008 is 68%, which is up from 49% in 1975–1977" (American Cancer Society, 2013). This indicates that "60% of 1-year cancer survivors experience clinically significant concerns about disease recurrence influencing the individual's functioning and quality of life" (American Cancer Society, 2014).

Survival from chronic health conditions brings new challenges for individuals throughout their lifespan, including lifelong and acute physical, psychological, and social adjustment difficulties. According to the American Childhood Cancer Organization (2013), "Two-thirds of those who survive the disease develop at least one chronic health condition that is classified as severe or life-threatening caused by late-effects of treatment. These effects often include heart damage, lung damage, infertility, cognitive impairment, growth deficits, hearing loss, and second cancers." Childhood

CBT for Psychological Well-Being in Cancer: A Skills Training Manual Integrating DBT, ACT, Behavioral Activation and Motivational Interviewing, First Edition. Mark Carlson.

cancer often results in lifelong disabilities, in addition to chronic health conditions. Because of this, cancer survivors are subject to ongoing monitoring across their lifespan. "Persons diagnosed with cancer will likely need physical and psychosocial care throughout their lives" (American Childhood Cancer Organization, 2013). "Patients and providers often are influenced by life circumstances and competing priorities, attitudes and beliefs about specific treatments, health literacy and understanding the health care system. These factors influence treatment compliance and overall cost" (American Cancer Society, 2014).

Health Care Costs

Cancer is linked with a wide range of illness, injuries, diseases, and mental health issues. "Cancer has been found to cause pain and the associated symptoms arising from a discrete cause, such as postoperative pain or pain associated with a malignancy. Millions suffer from acute or chronic pain every year and the effects of pain exact a tremendous cost on our country in health care costs, rehabilitation, and lost worker productivity, as well as the emotional and financial burden it places on Survivors and their families" (American Academy of Pain Medicine, 2015). According to a recent Institute of Medicine (IOM) report titled "Relieving Pain in America: A Blueprint for Transforming Prevention, Care, Education, and Research," "pain is a significant public health problem that costs society at least $560–$635 billion annually, an amount equal to about $2,000.00 for every person who lives in the United States. This includes the total incremental cost of health care due to pain ranging from $261–$300 billion and losses of productivity and associated issues ranging from $297–$336 billion. The costs of cancer can result in longer hospital stays, increased rates of re-hospitalization, increased emergency room visits, and a decreased ability to function that leads to lost income and insurance coverage. As such, Survivors' conditions often result in an inability to work and maintain health insurance, especially over the duration of their medical treatment."

"The financial costs of cancer are high for both the person with cancer and for society as a whole" (American Cancer Society, 2013). According to the National Institutes of Health (National Cancer Institute, 2015a), cancer "is a significant public health problem that costs society an estimated overall cost of $201.5 billion annually: $77.4 billion for direct medical costs (total of all health expenditures) and $124.0 billion for indirect mortality costs (cost of lost productivity due to premature death)." According to the American Cancer Society (2013), in 2006, the average cost of a single 30-day cancer drug prescription was $1,600; it is even higher today. Newer cancer treatments can cost as much as $10,000 for a month, and many protocols require more than a month of treatment. The American Cancer Society (2013) reports that "while those with health insurance face less worry regarding payment for treatment, those with no health insurance acquire extra worries when facing such an expensive disease. There is no guarantee that cancer expenses will be covered through insurance plans. Most personal bankruptcies that happen as a result of medical problems are filed by people who have health insurance."

Cancer and Functioning

A diagnosis of cancer causes distressing emotional experiences that decrease a person's ability to cope with their disease and treatment effectively. It is common for signs of impaired coping abilities to go unnoticed due to the severity and symptoms of the disease and treatment. Medical teams can assist patients in managing various side effects and symptoms, but patients may also benefit from mental health, social work, and counseling services to restore their quality of life and teach them coping skills (American Cancer Society, 2014). The American Cancer Society (2014) has found that 30–40% of patients have diagnosable mood disorders. Additionally, it suggests that psychological interventions can improve treatment adherence and patient–provider communication. Complete treatment adherence and improvements in communication between patients and their care teams were found to be correlated with low levels of depression and anxiety among cancer patients. Subpopulations at particular risk for elevated distress include racial/ethnic minorities, people diagnosed at younger ages, and those of lower socioeconomic status. These subpopulations have also been found to report greater difficulty regaining their quality of life in recovery. Distress is reported to negatively impact education and employment, at great cost to society (American Cancer Society, 2014).

The American Cancer Society (2014) states that "cancer patients experience pain at the time of diagnosis, during the course of active treatment, and after treatment has ended, even if their cancer does not return." Among cancer patients, pain is often underreported and undertreated. It has been found that 59% patients in active treatment report significant pain and about 33% of survivors report significant long-term pain post-treatment. Surgery, radiation therapy, and chemotherapy drugs can cause nerve damage. What manifests is chronic pain and a heightened risk of suicide among this population (American Cancer Society, 2014).

The comorbidity of mental health and physical problems resulting from pain is well established in research (Gatchel, 2004). Common comorbidity includes anxiety, depression, adjustment disorder, obsessive–compulsive disorder (OCD), histrionic personality disorder, and borderline personality disorder (BPD). The triggers are the pain and the uncertain prognosis of the diagnosed condition – specifically around progression of the disease, recurrence, reduced lifespan, end-of-life issues, treatment and side effects, cognitive, physical and behavioral impairments, and functional limitations (Ownsworth, 2009). Pain often results from chronic illness, injury, degeneration, and many related triggers in a chronic population. "People who experience chronic pain often experience a decrease in quality of life including: overall physical and emotional health, psychological and social well-being, fulfillment of personal expectations and goals, economic burden and financial stability, functional capacity to carry out daily routines, and activities of daily living. Additionally, destruction of family and social life, problems with treatment adherence and support systems, and decreased participation in sports or leisure activities have been found to increase the risk of clinical anxiety and depression, resulting in greater functional impairment and poor quality of life" (Pao & Weiner, 2011). This functional impairment and reduction in quality of life often leads to a variety of mental health concerns, including demoralization and a reduction in effective participation in treatment, as well as in life in general.

Cancer and Suicide

Cancer is often seen as a death sentence by mainstream society. Within the past decade, research has consistently demonstrated a strong correlation between cancer and suicide. In a survey of 2,924 cancer outpatients treated at one regional cancer center, 7.8% thought they would be "better off dead" or had considered hurting themselves in response to their diagnosis. While the general American population has a suicide rate of 10.6 out of every 100,000 persons per year, about 24 cancer patients out of every 100,000 complete suicide. Gender, prognosis, type of cancer, stage of disease, ethnicity, and family situation all contribute to suicide risk. Male cancer patients are nearly five times more likely to commit suicide than female patients, which remains consistent with suicide rates in the general population. Given the correlations, cancer patients may benefit from psychosocial support (Kendal & Kendal, 2012).

Medical Interventions

"Cancer is a group of diseases characterized by uncontrolled growth and spread of abnormal cells. Cancer can result in death, if the spread of abnormal cells is not controlled" (American Cancer Society, 2013). The American Cancer Society (2014) reports that cancer can be caused by both external factors (including tobacco, infectious organisms, chemicals, and radiation) and internal factors (including inherited mutations, hormones, immune conditions, and mutations that occur from metabolism). Together, these factors initiate or promote the development of cancer. The World Cancer Research Fund estimates that factors including obesity, physical inactivity, and poor nutrition will contribute to about one-quarter to one-third of new cancer cases expected to occur in the United States. Thus, with adequate lifestyle modification, cancer can be prevented.

A variety of medical interventions are frequently implemented in the treatment of cancer. The American Cancer Society (2013) reports that cancer is treated with surgery, radiation, chemotherapy, and hormone therapy. The recommendations for use vary based on cancer conditions. Attending to risk factors and engaging in regular medical screening tests that allow the detection and removal of precancerous growths can prevent cancer, but these procedures are costly. According to statistics provided by the National Cancer Institute (2010), 70% of cancer patients are treated with primary medical interventions of chemotherapy and radiation, and are subject to secondary medical interventions. By default, the majority of medical interventions used to treat cancer can result in costlier medical conditions among survivors. Bone and heart issues are two documented impairments. Many cancer treatments result in osteoporosis and heart damage due to reduced bone density and sustained high blood pressure. Increased risk of fractures and heart failure is associated with poorer quality of life among the general population; therapeutic interventions can improve these impairments among survivors (American Cancer Society, 2014).

Pharmacotherapy

Pharmacologic management is often included in the treatment regimen of cancer conditions; however, protocols vary according to individual differences, including the disease state and treatment response. The average cancer drug therapy costs over $100,000 per year (Sikora, 2004). Pharmacologic management of cancer tends to be unique and is tailored to the individual based on treatment response. Pain is comorbid with cancer. Pharmacotherapy for the treatment of pain includes the use of anticonvulsants, antidepressants, benzodiazepines, *N*-methyl-D-aspartate (NMDA) receptor antagonists, nonsteroidal anti-inflammatory drugs (NSAIDs), opioid therapy (e.g., oral, transdermal, transmucosal, internasal, and sublingual), skeletal muscle relaxants, and topical agents (American Society of Anesthesiologists, 2010).

Physical Therapy

The use of physical or restorative therapies for the treatment of chronic pain caused by cancer has been popular. A review of available research on the use of physical or restorative therapies conducted by the American Society of Anesthesiologists (2010) indicated promising results. Randomized controlled trials (RCTs) that incorporated a variety of these therapies, including fitness classes, exercise therapy, and physiotherapy, were effective in treating low back pain. American Society of Anesthesiologists and American Society of Regional Anesthesia members recommended that physical or restorative therapies be implemented in the treatment strategy for patients with low back pain and other chronic pain conditions. Additionally, restorative therapies may be beneficial in restoring function lost due to the cancer itself.

Palliative Care

Palliative care is care given to improve the quality of life of patients who have a serious or life-threatening disease, such as cancer. The goal of palliative care is to prevent or treat, as early as possible, the symptoms and side effects of the disease and its treatment, in addition to any related psychological, social, and spiritual problems. The goal is not to cure. Palliative care is also called "comfort care," "supportive care," and "symptom management" (National Cancer Institute, 2015a).

Integrated Behavioral Health

Integrated medical care will require more than just "integrating" mental health and behavioral health clinicians into the existing health care team of physician, nurse practitioner, nurse, physical therapist, and nutritionist: it will require "integrated behavioral health," meaning that behavioral health clinicians must provide "integrated" services that combine and integrate individual and family dynamics and individual and family or systemic interventions. The need for behavioral health is important because about 50% of all patients in primary care present with psychological comorbidities, and 60% of psychological or psychiatric disorders are treated in primary care settings (Pirl et al., 2001).

A major meta-analysis of 91 studies published between 1967 and 1997 provided evidence for what researchers call the "medical cost-offset effect." Behavioral health interventions, including various forms of psychotherapy, were provided to medical patients with a history of overutilization, as well as to patients being treated for only psychological disorders, such as substance abuse. Average savings resulting from the implementation of psychological interventions were estimated to be about 20% (Chiles et al., 1999). In short, the medical cost-offset effect occurs when emotionally distressed medical patients receive appropriate behavioral health treatment. As a result of this treatment, they tend to reduce their utilization of all forms of medical care. Even though there is a cost associated with behavioral health treatment, the overall cost savings is considerable.

Clinical Implications of Integrated Behavioral Health

The emerging integrated health care philosophy is that integrated behavioral health care will utilize behavioral interventions for a wide range of health and mental health concerns. The primary focus will be on resolving problems within the primary care setting, as well as on engaging in health promotion and compliance enhancement for "at-risk" patients. The goal of health care integration is to position the behavioral health counselor to support the physician or other primary care provider and bring more specialized knowledge to problems that require additional help.

Accordingly, the behavioral health counselor's role will be to identify the problem, target treatment, and manage medical patients with psychological problems using a behavioral approach. They will help patients replace maladaptive behaviors with more adaptive ones. In addition, they will use psychoeducation and client education strategies to provide skills training.

More specifically, the behavioral health counselor will be expected to provide expertise in dealing with undermotivated, noncompliant, or otherwise resistant patients. They will utilize motivational interviewing (MI) with individual patients (Rollnick et al., 2008) and with patients' families to increase readiness for change. They will also utilize focused cognitive behavioral strategies to increase compliance with treatment regimens, reduce symptoms, and increase acceptance of chronic and life-threatening illnesses (Sperry, 2006).

Cognitive Behavioral Therapy

Cancer has a significant impact on patients' lives and on the support systems around them. Adult cancer patients and their family members suffer from traumatic psychological distress, and psychological interventions may be beneficial (Butler et al.,

2006; Han et al., 2005; Koopman et al., 2002). Cognitive factors play an important role in the experience of cancer (Gatchel et al., 2007). Group therapy, using cognitive behavioral therapy (CBT), has been found to be successful in treating anxiety and depression among those diagnosed with cancer (Edelman et al., 1999; Monga et al., 2009). Clinical insight suggests that group therapy can be an effective intervention for parents of this population, and can decrease anxiety (Edelman et al., 1999; Gilder et al., 1978; Mitchell et al., 2006).

According to Gatchel et al. (2007), CBT interventions are based on the view that an individual's beliefs, evaluation, and interpretation of their health condition, in addition to their pain, disability, and coping abilities, will impact the degree of both physical and emotional disability of the disease condition. Currently, CBT-based techniques vary widely in the literature; they can include distraction, imagery, motivational self-talk, relaxation training, biofeedback, development of coping strategies, goal setting, and changing maladaptive beliefs about pain and disease.

It is common for cancer patients to experience acute and chronic pain. Morely et al. (1999) conducted a meta-analysis of randomized trials of CBT in the treatment of chronic pain. They concluded that the use of CBT treatment to replace maladaptive patient cognitions and behaviors with more adaptive ones is effective for a variety of pain conditions. More recently, Linton & Nordin (2006) reported a 5-year follow-up of an RCT of CBT intervention for clients suffering from chronic back pain. They found that CBT interventions (compared to the control group) resulted in significantly less pain, a more active life, higher perceived quality of life, and better overall health. In addition, significant economic benefits were associated with the clients who had completed CBT treatment.

Scope of the Book

Psychological interventions are supportive and typically ancillary in nature for most cancer patients. There are many individuals who have exhausted their options for primary medical interventions and are faced with the challenge of having pain and disease as a part of their lives, with little or no hope for positive change or a cure. Demoralization is a common reaction to this reality. The field of psychology has few treatment manuals and integrated treatment options for clients as they move through the process of finding a cure, or learning to live with disease. One of the goals of this book is to provide practitioners with one of the first comprehensive manuals for the treatment of cancer patients, which can be applied across modalities and levels of care.

Chapter 3

Introduction to the TAG Concept for Group and/or Individual Therapy

The TAG Concept for Cancer and Psychological Well-Being

Therapists are encouraged to adopt the TAG (Teach, Apply, and Generalize) concept (Carlson, 2014) when in session with individuals. I am often asked by clinicians across the United States, "How do we know when we are doing effective work?" I consistently answer that we need to be **Teaching** skills and approaches, have patients **Apply** these skills and approaches during session, and **Generalize** what is learned to their lives outside of the therapeutic session, while tracking outcomes. The TAG concept has its roots in the philosophy of contextualism. Leaders in contextualism include James, Dewey, Mead, K. Burke, and Bormann. The predominant character of behavior analysis – or, at least, what is central and distinctive about behavior analysis – is contextualistic (Hayes, 1998). The philosophy of contextualism corresponds well with behavioral analytic concepts of the operant, accomplishment of attainable goals, the active role of the therapist, and working with order and randomness. The TAG concept incorporates these key aspects into its fundamental structure and operations. TAG is based on CBT through practice, primary intervention strategies, and skills training. It incorporates skills and core components of: dialectical behavior therapy (DBT), MI, acceptance and commitment therapy (ACT), and behavioral activation (BA). Grief and loss work, existential approaches, mindfulness, and identity development are also incorporated. The manual is written from the perspective of evidence-based practice in psychology (EBPP): the integration of the best available research with clinical expertise in the context of patient characteristics, culture, and preferences (American Psychological Association, 2015).

There are many theories and approaches in the field of psychology. In developing TAG, empirically supported treatments (ESTs) were identified and relevant research was reviewed. It was decided to continue its development through a contextual model that incorporates components shared by all approaches to psychotherapy, as well as six

CBT for Psychological Well-Being in Cancer: A Skills Training Manual Integrating DBT, ACT, Behavioral Activation and Motivational Interviewing, First Edition. Mark Carlson.
© 2017 John Wiley & Sons, Ltd. Published 2017 by John Wiley & Sons, Ltd.

elements that are common to the rituals and procedures used by all psychotherapists. Arkowitz (1992) suggests that dissatisfaction with individual theoretical approaches spawned three movements: (i) theoretical integration, (ii) technical eclecticism, and (iii) common factors. The contextual model is a derivative of the common factors view (Wampold, 2001).

According to Wampold (2001):

> A contextual model was proposed by Jerome Frank in his book, *Persuasion and Healing* (Frank & Frank, 1991). According to Frank and Frank (1991), "the aim of psychotherapy is to help people feel and function better by encouraging appropriate modifications in their assumptive worlds, thereby transforming the meanings of experiences to more favorable ones" (p. 30). Persons who present for psychotherapy are demoralized and have a variety of problems, typically depression and anxiety. That is, people seek psychotherapy for the demoralization that results from their symptoms rather than from symptom relief. Frank has proposed that "psychotherapy achieves its effects largely and directly by treating demoralization and only indirectly treating overt symptoms of covert psychopathology"...

Frank & Frank (1991) describe the components shared by all approaches to psychotherapy. The first component is an emotionally charged, confiding relationship with a helping person (i.e., the therapist). The second component is that the context of the relationship is a healing setting, in which the client presents to a professional whom they believe can provide help and who is entrusted to work on their behalf. The third component is a rationale, conceptual scheme, or myth that provides a plausible explanation for the patient's symptoms and prescribes a ritual or procedure for resolving them. The final component is a ritual or procedure based on the rationale (i.e., believed to be a viable means of helping the client), which requires the active participation of both client and therapist.

Frank & Frank (1991) discuss six elements that are common to the rituals and procedures used by all psychotherapists. First, the therapist combats the client's sense of alienation by developing a relationship that is maintained after the client divulges feelings of demoralization. Second, the therapist maintains the patient's expectation of being helped by linking hope for improvement to the process of therapy. Third, the therapist provides new learning experiences. Fourth, the client's emotions are aroused as a result of the therapy. Fifth, the therapist enhances the client's sense of mastery or self-efficacy. Sixth, the therapist provides opportunities for practice.

Wampold (2001) furthers this concept by adding that in the contextual model, specific ingredients are necessary to construct a coherent treatment that therapists have faith in and that provides a convincing rationale to clients.

The Biopsychosocial Model

This manual is written using a biopsychosocial model of treatment. The American Psychological Association defines the **biopsychosocial model** as: a model of health and illness that suggests that links among the nervous system, the immune system, behavioral styles, cognitive processing, and environmental factors can put people at risk of illness. The biopsychosocial model is an extension of the biomedical model

(Sperry, 2006) that incorporates psychological and sociocultural dimensions with the biomedical dimension. The biopsychosocial model fosters integrative care and is the operative model in the practice of behavioral health (Sperry, 2014).

Developing a Program through the TAG Concept

Many clinicians will choose to infuse the contents of this manual into their existing practice. There is a large need among individuals diagnosed with cancer and mental health issues for more structured and intensive services. The TAG concept can easily be adapted to create a program and serve as the foundation of a service delivery model.

The TAG program was created for individuals experiencing issues with comorbid mental health and cancer. It is designed to be 3–6 months in duration, or more, and to have flexibility in implementation across modalities of treatment. The concepts and skills training of the TAG program can be easily applied in individual therapy if that is the primary modality for intervention. The individual therapist will be able to modify the format and select concepts and skill sets to customize for the individual. Such modification relies on the education, training, and expertise of the clinician, since it deviates from the initial design and intensity of the program.

The design that will initially be discussed is a group skills training model. Groups meet two times weekly for 3 hours. A clinician does not need to adhere to a specific order for the sessions. The structure of the program provides the clinician a high degree of flexibility. This allows for individualization and customization of the skills and concepts to each individual in the group. Each session is formatted to have goals for each individual and for the group as a whole. There are multiple discussion topics, designed to assess each individual's strengths and barriers to effective functioning, and to establish a baseline of understanding and coping. The discussion points can also provide a general orientation and segue to the coping skills. Each session has general coping concepts and specific skill sets for each individual to learn. The individual is taught a set of skills, encouraged to practice in the session, and then told to generalize the skills to multiple aspects of their lives through problem solving.

Group/Session Structure

The group structure of the TAG program is designed to meet twice a week for 3 hours. Each hour is designed to have a specific focus for each individual and for the group as a whole.

Section 1: teaching

The teaching section is prioritized as the first section of the day, to provide grounding for each individual, to establish expectations that all members will be focusing on learning and applying skills, and to reinforce participation throughout the process. This section is designed to be 45–50 minutes in length.

The first part of this section introduces the specific goals for the teaching. It starts with an introduction to the topic and an explanation of why the topic is challenging for individuals. Each individual is engaged in the process, to identify whether this is a strength area for them or a barrier to more effective functioning. If an individual identifies the topic as a strength area, they are encouraged to establish a goal of building consistency and a sense of mastery with the skills. If an individual identifies it as a barrier to more effective functioning, they are encouraged to establish a goal of learning the core concepts of the skill sets, create an initial plan, and commit to practice the skills in session. Individuals who are working toward building consistency and mastery may then serve as mentors to those who are newer to the skill sets. Once the individuals and the group as a whole have set goals, the general topic is discussed from a variety of perspectives. This allows for engagement in the process, general orientation to the topic, and establishment of baselines of functioning. Individuals are encouraged to provide examples from their lives as to why and how the topic is relevant. The clinician is encouraged to identify strengths, barriers to effective functioning, and needs, and to provide a segue to the specific skill sets to be taught. This part is designed to be highly interactive and organic in its process. This is where members discuss the topic's relevancy to their situation and see that they are not isolated in their experience as other members are encouraged to share. This provides a direct grounding experience for many individuals and "normalizes" their reality.

The next part of the teaching section is the skills training component. This is the core of the TAG program. Each session has multiple skill sets to teach. The curriculum is designed to have multiple skill sets that work directly with the current topic and have generalizability to global coping. This is intended to ground the individual in their current needs, strengths, coping strategies, and global functioning. The next step is to teach specific sets of cognitive and behavioral skills and concepts designed to increase each individual's functioning and/or quality of life. The skill sets are focused on the current topic and how the individual can learn and apply the skills directly in the session. Each individual incorporates a set of skills into their identified goal work and commits to a plan to generalize the skills into their daily functioning. This plan is then reviewed in the third part, where it is problem solved to address the individual's strengths and barriers.

Section 2: application

The application section is designed to focus on pattern recognition and awareness (based on the principles of self-monitoring and adherence to treatment). This section is designed to be 45–50 minutes in length. A tracking card or diary card is the primary tool used. Each individual completes their tracking card before the session, and reviews it with the clinician and the entire group. The card includes areas of functioning, needs, strengths, skills used/attempted, and how effective the individual's application of skills has been since the last session. Peers provide feedback in the form of support, challenge, and suggestions to increase the effective application and generalizability of the skill sets. Treatment goals and objectives are also reviewed daily in this section.

Section 3: generalization (problem solving)

The problem-solving section is designed to assist individuals in applying their strengths to overcoming barriers to effective coping. This section is designed to be 45–50 minutes in length. Each individual is expected to identify one goal area that they want to focus on. They take problem-solving time to discuss their strengths, difficulties, skill implementation plan, and commitment to skill use, and to receive feedback from the clinician and their peers on their action plan. The goal of this section is to have the individual commit to applying their skills outside of the therapeutic setting, create a clear action plan designed to increase the efficacy of their coping strategies (incorporating new skills that have been taught in the program), and establish a review/completion time before the next session. The completed action plan will be reviewed in Section 2 of the next group session. This increases the individual's accountability for follow-through and establishes continuity between sessions.

Curriculum Overview

The manual starts with seven sessions to orient the clinician to the population, the methodology, and the proposed approach. This provides the clinician with the necessary tools to integrate this manual into their existing practice, or to create an entire program with the manual as a foundation.

    The curriculum is designed to be topic-driven (arranged by topic) in an open group format. Therapy is multimodal, incorporating group and individual therapy. The program is organized through the biopsychosocial model. There are seven sessions targeting coping with the biological aspects of mental health and cancer, seven sessions targeting coping with the psychological aspects of mental health and cancer, and seven sessions targeting coping with the social aspects of mental health and cancer. The term "individual" is used in place of "patient" or "client" to challenge stigma labeling. Personalizing therapeutic approaches leads to adherence, ownership of the process, and personal responsibility.

Sources and recommended readings

It is recommended that the clinician review the original publications and material in the References section of the book for further conceptual depth and understanding.

General curriculum

Seven sessions form the focus of orienting the clinician to the manual's approach. This section includes:

1. Orienting the individual to therapy
2. Skills training
3. Interventions and strategies
4. Safety assessment and contracting
5. Cognitive and behavioral analysis

6. Self-regulation and illness perceptions
7. Chronic illness

Biological curriculum

Seven sessions form the focus of skills training designed to target issues related to the biological nature of the individual's mental health and cancer. This section includes:

1. Increased functioning and quality of life
2. Goal setting and motivation
3. Orientation to change
4. Working with your team
5. Adherence to treatment protocols
6. Pain
7. Healthy habits and sleep

Psychological curriculum

Seven sessions form the focus of skills training designed to target issues related to the psychological nature of the individual's mental health and cancer. This section includes:

1. Anxiety
2. Depression
3. Trauma and retraumatization
4. Increasing resiliency through stress management
5. Anger management
6. Finding meaning
7. Stigma

Social curriculum

Seven sessions form the focus of skills training designed to target issues related to the social nature of the individual's mental health and cancer. This section includes:

1. Intimacy
2. Problem solving
3. Nurturing support systems
4. Managing conflict
5. Demoralization and remoralization
6. Styles of interacting
7. Grief and loss

Goals of the Program

The goals of the program are to reduce hospitalizations and emergency room visits, decrease unneeded doctor visits, improve individual functioning, improve quality of life, restore hope and activity, decrease demoralization while increasing resiliency through stress management, and reduce overall cost of care for the targeted population.

Suggested Program/Treatment Outcome Measures

Partners for Change Outcomes Management System

The Partners for Change Outcome Management System (PCOMS) is a well-researched, quality-improvement strategy that boils down to partnering with clients to identify those who aren't responding to clinician business as usual and addressing the lack of progress in a proactive way that keeps clients engaged while therapists collaboratively seek new directions. Five RCTs conducted by the clinical developer, Dr. Barry Duncan, and researchers at the Heart and Soul of Change Project have shown PCOMS to significantly improve effectiveness in real clinical settings, as well as to substantially reduce costs related to length of treatment and provider productivity. Because of these RCTs, PCOMS is recognized in the Substance Abuse Mental Health Services Administration's (SAMHSA) National Registry of Evidence-based Programs and Practices. PCOMS has been implemented by hundreds of organizations in all 50 states and in 20 countries.

PCOMS uses two four-item scales to solicit consumer feedback regarding factors proven to predict success regardless of treatment model or presenting problem: client assessment of early progress (using the outcome rating scale, ORS) and the quality of the alliance or match with the provider (using the session rating scale, SRS).

PCOMS:

- Provides objective, quantifiable data on the effectiveness of providers and systems of care
- Uses measures that are valid and reliable, but feasible for each clinical encounter
- Provides a methodology for consumer preferences to guide choice of intervention

Consequently, unlike other methods of measuring outcome, this system truly assigns consumers key roles in determining how services are delivered, while honoring the time demands of frontline clinical work and documenting proof of value (Duncan & Reese, 2012; www.heartandsoulofchange.com).

Outcome and Session Rating Scales

The ORS and SRS are brief measures for tracking client functioning and the quality of the therapeutic alliance. Each instrument takes less than a minute for consumers to complete and for clinicians to score and interpret. Both scales were developed in clinical settings where longer, research-oriented measures had been deemed impractical for routine use. Versions of the ORS and SRS are available for adults, children, adolescents, and groups in 18 different languages. Individual clinicians may download the scales free of charge after registering online at www.scottdmiller.com. A significant and growing body of research shows the scales to be valid, reliable, and feasible for assessing progress and the alliance across a wide range of consumers and presenting concerns (Miller & Bergmann, 2012).

Treatment Outcome Package

The treatment outcome package (TOP) is an outcome measure used to track changes in psychological symptoms and functional domains over the course of treatment. It was developed by Kraus, Seligman, and Jordan as a comprehensive outcome measurement tool for use in naturalistic settings that could gather information about the full spectrum of presenting problems and psychopathology (www.outcomereferrals.com). Additionally, the TOP collects data about extraneous variables (e.g., changes in medications, medical illnesses, major life changes, etc.) that serve as risk factors with the potential to significantly influence the course of treatment for behavioral health clients (Kraus and colleagues have named these "case-mix variables"). The TOP is designed to maximize the chances of measuring meaningful changes in psychological symptoms, functional domains, and case-mix variables over the course of treatment.

The TOP was normed on a large sample of adults with a variety of disorders seeking treatment in a variety of behavioral health services. It generates reports using 12 clinically relevant scales that assist clinicians with (i) diagnosis, (ii) treatment planning, (iii) outcome assessment, and (iv) improving the therapeutic relationship. These scales are: depression, quality of life, psychosis, panic, violence, work functioning, mania, sleep, substance abuse, social conflict, sexual functioning, and suicidality (www.outcomereferrals.com).

SF-36

The SF-36 is a short-form survey that was designed to evaluate health status as part of the Medical Outcomes Study. Initially formed and validated in 1988, it was revised in 1996, and it has been cited in several thousand publications. It provides scores on a scale from 0 to 100 in eight different domains: physical functioning, role-physical, bodily pain, general health, vitality, social functioning, role-emotional, and mental health. The reliability of these eight scales and subsequent summary measures has been evaluated in studies using internal consistency and test–retest methodology, obtaining a minimum of .70 in the reliability coefficient in all but a few studies, with .80 or higher being standard. The validity of this assessment is supported by various studies indicating that the measure has content, concurrent, criterion, construct, and predictive validity. The SF-36 v1.0 is available for free from the RAND Corporation, and the SF-36 v2.0 is currently controlled and licensed by Quality Metric (www.rand.org).

Quality of Life Questionnaire

The Quality of Life Questionnaire is an assessment tool designed by David Evans and Wendy Cope in 1983 (first published for public use in 1989). Its purpose is to measure "the relationship between a client's quality of life and other behaviors or afflictions, such as physical health, psychological health, and alcohol or other substance use" (Multi-Health Systems, 2012). It contains a total of 192 true/false items, is self-administered, and takes about half an hour to complete. It can be scored by the administrator, and results are provided through five domains (with a total of 15 subdomains): general well-being, interpersonal relationship, organizational activity, occupational activity, and leisure/recreational activity. It has been used or referenced in approximately 600 studies, and several psychometric evaluations have been conducted to support its validity and reliability. It is available for purchase from Multi-Health Systems and has manual and Web-based scoring options (Multi-Health Systems, 2012).

Behavioral Assessment of Pain Questionnaire

The Behavioral Assessment of Pain Questionnaire (BAP-2) is a self-administered, multidimensional assessment tool for understanding factors that may be working to exacerbate and/or maintain sub-acute and chronic nonmalignant pain. The BAP-2 was developed with a normative chronic pain sample of over 1,000 individuals suffering from sub-acute and chronic pain. As a pain-assessment instrument, the BAP-2 has been shown to have good reliability and validity data (Lewandowski, 2006).

The BAP-2 was developed using a biopsychosocial approach and examines various pain characteristics (e.g., pain intensity, pain behavior, pain descriptions), past and current levels of physical activity, activity avoidance levels, fears of pain and reinjury, mood, attitudes and beliefs about pain, and behavioral responses to pain. It has over 32 scales, which measure such variables as the impact that significant others – such as physicians and family members – may have on the individual's current pain behavior, and makes appropriate recommendations for successful treatment.

The BAP-2 generates a clinical profile report that helps the treating clinician develop a unique treatment plan tailored for the individual. An overall estimate of dysfunction and impairment is estimated for each individual compared to the normative sample (Lewandowski, 2006).

Symptom Checklist-90-R

The Symptom Checklist-90-R (SCL-90-R) (Pearson, 1994) instrument helps evaluate a broad range of psychological problems and symptoms of psychopathology. The instrument is also useful in measuring patient progress and treatment outcomes.

The SCL-90-R is used by clinical psychologists, psychiatrists, and professionals in mental health, medical, and educational settings, as well as for research purposes. It can be useful in the initial evaluation of patients at intake as an objective method of symptom assessment, in measuring patient progress during and after treatment to monitor change, as an outcomes measurement for treatment programs and providers through aggregated patient information, and in helping measure changes in symptoms such as depression and anxiety in clinical trials.

The SCL-90-R test contains only 90 items and can be completed in just 12–15 minutes. The test helps measure nine primary symptom dimensions and is designed to provide an overview of a patient's symptoms, and their intensity, at a specific point in time. The progress report graphically displays patient progress over up to five previous administrations, by providing an index of symptom severity. The assessment helps facilitate treatment decisions and identify patients before problems become acute. The Global Severity Index can be used as a summary of the test. More than 1,000 studies have been conducted, demonstrating the reliability, validity, and utility of the instrument.

Symptom scales include: somatization, obsessive–compulsive, interpersonal sensitivity, depression, anxiety, hostility, phobic anxiety, paranoid ideation, and psychoticism.

Illness Perception Questionnaire

Research using a variety of different assessment techniques suggests patients cluster their ideas about an illness around five coherent themes or components: identity (the label of the illness and the symptoms the patient views as being part of it), cause (personal ideas about etiology, which may include simple single causes or more complex multiple causal models), timeline (how long the patient believes the illness will last, categorized as acute, chronic, or episodic), consequences (expected effects and outcomes), and cure/control (how the patient will recover from or control the illness) (www.uib.no/ipq/). These components provide a framework that allows patients to make sense of their symptoms, assess health risk, and direct action and coping. Each component holds a perception about one aspect of the illness, and together they provide the individual's coherent view of the illness as a whole.

Chapter 4
Clinical Manual

General Curriculum

Session focus: Orienting the individual to therapy

TAG
Teach – Apply – Generalize

- The goal of this session is to:
  - o Establish inclusionary/exclusionary criteria
  - o Identify the modality or modalities of treatment
  - o Identify the level of care (LOC) that is needed
  - o Prepare orientation materials for individuals
- What to discuss:
  - o The assessment process
  - o Informed consent to treatment
  - o Orientation to the approach
  - o The structure of the sessions/program
- Skills to teach:
  - o Relevant forms and procedures
- Generalize:
  - o Discuss goodness of fit or potential referrals

Orienting the individual to therapy

Introduction of the topic
This session is designed to orient the clinician to the proposed therapeutic structure and process. It is important to consider what community resources are available and what the needs of the target population are when designing your service delivery model. You might want to start a full program or to infuse this work into your existing practice. There are a few important aspects to account for in this process.

CBT for Psychological Well-Being in Cancer: A Skills Training Manual Integrating DBT, ACT, Behavioral Activation and Motivational Interviewing, First Edition. Mark Carlson.
© 2017 John Wiley & Sons, Ltd. Published 2017 by John Wiley & Sons, Ltd.

Medical necessity, LOC, and treatment modalities

There are many factors to consider when establishing medical necessity. The basic consideration is whether the individual will reasonably benefit from the proposed service in accordance with federal, state, and managed care organization (MCO) guidelines. Once medical necessity for the individual (or the program itself through contracts) is established, the LOC needs to be addressed. Individuals have a wide range of need. The frequency and duration of sessions may need to be scheduled with fluidity. It is important to be consistent in your approach when scheduling sessions or meeting times. The individual's needs will likely vary over the course of treatment. This manual is designed to be adaptable to changes in the frequency and duration of the therapeutic work in what is a very volatile and changing population.

Treatment modalities are also a core consideration. Typical modalities include both individual and group therapy. Individual therapy can range from multiple times weekly during times of crisis to a more infrequent monthly schedule, which tends to be more maintenance-oriented. Group therapy can have a very wide range as well, from daily contact (as in a partial hospital setting) to once monthly (as commonly seen in aftercare services). The clinician will need to understand the populations to be treated and their needs, and to design programming accordingly. Fortunately, there are many options available. Health care in the United States is moving toward more integrated models of service delivery, which is making establishing the need for services, gaining contracts with payers, and being reimbursed for services more of a norm.

Inclusionary/exclusionary criteria

The clinician needs to establish who will potentially benefit from therapeutic services. When a specialty service such as this is being considered, it is imperative to establish the populations for which it may be beneficial. This approach is designed to treat individuals experiencing mental health issues who also have a diagnosis of cancer. The clinician will have to assess the appropriateness of the individual for this approach. The following list can be used as a guide to assist in the assessment process.

Is the individual able to engage in therapy in a meaningful manner when considering:

- **Medical stability** – Is the individual medically stable or currently compromised in some way?
- **Anticipated course of the illness** – When is the right time for the individual to start psychological services?
- **Availability to consistently attend programming** – Consider medical stability, medical appointment frequencies, and transportation
- **Primary mental health diagnosis** – Does the individual demonstrate medical and mental health comorbidities?
- **Type and stage of illness** – Is the individual newly diagnosed, receiving ongoing treatment, a survivor, in remission, or end-of-life?
- **History of treatment** – Is the individual new to psychological services?
- **Medical necessity for services** – Does the individual need your services, and at what LOC?

- **Readiness for change** – Is the individual ready to do the work, or are they contemplating the need?
- **Cognitive abilities** – Consider tracking, attention and concentration, and memory, which can all be compromised by medical procedures.

Special considerations for group therapy:

- **Open/closed group** – Is the group run in discrete sections or in an ongoing manner?
- **Homogeneous/heterogeneous populations** – Consider culture, age, socioeconomic status, gender, and other variables
- **Types/stages of illness** – This is the strongest area for group cohesion. Groups may work best if they are separated into four categories: newly diagnosed, receiving active medical interventions, remission, and end-of-life. A case can also be made for diversity in types and stages.
- **Personality structure/disorders** – Group therapy may be counterindicated in this population for individuals experiencing psychosis or with narcissistic personality disorder. This needs to be assessed on a case-by-case basis.

Preparing orientation materials

It is important to have materials prepared at the start of therapy. This assists in the orientation process, by answering many of the questions individuals will have. The materials I suggest are the Bill of Rights for Persons Served, an outline of the program itself or a one-page description of individual therapy, rules and expectations, attendance contracts, safety contracts, the program handouts from this manual (**Group Rules/Expectations, Attendance Discharge Contract, Safety Contract**), and other materials relevant to the services being provided. Individuals find it helpful if you allow time to review the materials in session and address any questions they may have. If any of the forms provided in this manual do not meet your needs or the needs of your consumers, you will need to modify them.

- **Group Rules/Expectations** – This form is given to all participants during the orientation process. They are encouraged to ask questions and discuss areas that may be of concern for them. All answers and discussions surround the need for a safe and consistent environment in which to work.
- **Attendance/Discharge Contract** – This form is given to all participants during the orientation process. They are encouraged to address any and all scheduling concerns that they may have. If an individual is not able to commit to the attendance requirements, I suggest that you consider delaying their start in therapy until they can meet the commitments. The attendance contract is designed to promote consistency for all involved in the treatment process.
- **Safety Contract** – This form is given to all participants during the orientation process. They are oriented to all safety requirements, policies, and procedures.

Teaching skills (T)

This session is not designed to be skills training. It outlines the process for establishing programming and orienting individuals to the approach.

Applying skills and concepts (A)

- Complete the assessment process
- Provide orientation materials such as program handouts, a description of services, **Group Rules/Expectations**, an **Attendance/Discharge Contract**, and a **Safety Contract**

Generalizing skills and concepts (G)

- Assign the individual the task of reviewing the orientation materials and prepare for the next session
- Problem-solve barriers to this process

Notes to clinicians and individuals

- The process of orientation starts with the first contact with the individual and ends with their discharge. It is an ongoing and dynamic process.
- Clinicians have difficult decisions to make when establishing criteria for planned programming. There are many factors to consider, including community resources and needs, client variables, contracting, funding, training, supervision, space, and coordination of care.
- I typically provide a three-ring binder to all individuals, which includes the previously mentioned forms, handouts from the manual, paper for taking notes, and a printed schedule of all of their sessions.
- You may want to question the practice of providing group and individual therapy to the same individual from the same clinician. There are times where there are no other options, but it can present unique challenges.
- Part of orientation is identifying that an individual is the "leader" of their treatment team. This empowers the individual, while putting the responsibility for self-advocacy and self-regulation on them.

Session focus: Skills training

TAG
Teach – Apply – Generalize

- The goal of this session is to:
  - Orient the clinician to skills training
- Basic assumptions about the individual
- Common questions about skills training

Skills training

Introduction of the topic
This session is designed to orient the clinician to skills training based around promoting increased functioning and quality of life for individuals seeking treatment.

According to Gatchel (2004), "the major goal of Cognitive Behavioral Therapy (CBT) is to replace maladaptive coping skills, cognitions, emotions and behaviors with more adaptive ones." Turk & Flor (2006) describe CBT as having six phases: (i) assessment, (ii) reconceptualization, (iii) skills acquisition, (iv) skills consolidation, (v) generalization and maintenance, and (vi) post-treatment assessment and follow-up. Briefly, assessment measures the degree of impairment and sets the stage for course of treatment. Reconceptualization challenges maladaptive thought patterns. Skills acquisition teaches skills to address daily challenges in the individual's life. Skills consolidation and application uses homework to reinforce the skills the individual is learning. Generalization and maintenance helps externalize skill use outside of the therapeutic session for current and future needs. Post-treatment assessment and follow-up is for monitoring the skills applications to the individual's life. Turk and Flor's phase model provides a clear framework for the TAG concept.

Basic assumptions about individuals
There are a few basic assumptions to consider when engaging in skills training, which serve as a guide and ongoing orientation for the clinician.

Belief in the client's desire and inherent capacity to grow and change
When individuals are doing well, they create beliefs and behavioral strategies to maintain their functioning and quality of life. When they start to struggle or challenges are presented, their maintenance strategies do not apply effectively and they need new strategies oriented toward adaptation and survival. Once stability is achieved, there can be a return toward maintenance, but individuals may not return to the stable state in which they existed before they experienced their physical and mental health challenges.

Acceptance/self-acceptance as a prerequisite to change
A quote from Carl Rogers summarizes this point quite well: "The curious paradox is that when I accept myself just as I am, then I can change." Acceptance provides a

starting point for the individual. If one rejects their situation or their experience, one is not grounded in the reality of one's own experience. As a byproduct, there may not be a clear delineation of one's needs, wants, or desires. This grounding is needed to provide a framework for therapy, and is the basis of assessment and treatment planning.

Empathic understanding of the client's internal frame of reference (i.e., validation)

Individuals need to be validated in order to build a trusting therapeutic alliance. They need to know that the clinician is listening and attempting to connect with their experience. This connection allows for vulnerability, growth, and trust to be a part of the course of therapy.

Non-judgmental, unconditional positive regard

Many individuals fear the possibility of judgment on the part of the clinician. It is important to create a therapeutic atmosphere based on safety. Few individuals will take positive risks in therapy if judgment is present.

Congruence: authenticity and genuineness on the part of the therapist (disclosure in the interest of therapy)

Many clinicians use self-disclosure in therapy. A good rule of thumb is to have all disclosure have therapeutic value for the individual. This also allows the clinician to provide feedback in session on how they are responding to the topic, the process, and the relationship itself. It can give the individual challenges/support in regards to their thoughts and behaviors. Some clinicians refer to this as the "reality-check" process, as they are telling the client what they need to hear.

Present focus (versus past or future)

It is important to orient the individual to their current experience in order to effectively engage in skills training. Individuals can learn from the past, which commonly serves as a guide for learning through the consequences of what has been done. The future can be addressed by challenging ineffective cognitive patterns involving denial, catastrophizing, minimizing, and anticipated possible outcomes. Problem-solving strategies and skills-oriented action plans are created in session and linked to the individual's life through homework and generalizing strategies.

Entering the relationship through the client's reality

Skills training starts with the individual's reality. This is a challenge for many clinicians, as they commonly focus on change and the need for change. There are times where clinicians push too quickly or impose change that is not driven by the individual. This is a reminder to slow the process down and focus on where the client is at, not where they "should be." Explore their experience in order to gather information that can assist in guiding the therapeutic process.

Clients are doing their best: behaviors meet needs

It can serve as a healthy reminder to consider that individuals are doing their best with their current attempts to cope. No matter how extreme their behaviors, they have met or are currently meeting needs. Assess what needs are being addressed and how the behaviors do and do not work for all involved, and then address how the individual might be more effective in their attempts at needs attainment.

Common questions about skills training
Skills training can be a very dynamic and individualized process in both group and individual therapy. When the clinician is engaged and motivated by the material and the process, the individual tends to respond in a very active manner. Here are some of the common questions clinicians ask:

Do I teach skills in a specific order?
This can be an effective strategy. Many skills-training approaches organize sets of skills into groups designed to target specific aspects of functioning. This can provide a logical progression based upon the content, structure, and goals of the skill sets themselves. DBT provides a nice example. Individual skills are typically grouped into modules of teachings, such as emotion regulation, distress tolerance, interpersonal effectiveness, and mindfulness (Linehan, 1993). Each module has sets of skills to promote healthy functioning, which can be taught in a stepwise and sequential manner. They can also be taught by combining skills from each of the modules in order to address a specific topic, need, or aspect of functioning. The important point is to individualize the skills that are being taught to the individual seeking services.

How do I individualize the approach?
This can be done in a variety of ways. The most common is to identify a topic that is relevant to the individual and begin a discussion from there. Identify the needs/wants of the individual, assess their strengths, identify barriers to effective functioning, and introduce skills that can promote more effective functioning. Review their treatment plan and the agreed-upon goals and objectives to create and maintain a clear course for treatment. Incorporate all assessments and tracking tools directly into treatment sessions and the treatment planning process. The skills components can be taught in a proactive manner to create healthy habits over time or in a reactive manner to address distressing events.

Is there a suggested structure for individual therapy sessions and skills training?
There is no right way to structure therapy sessions; it is more about finding what works for the individual. One suggested approach is to start the session with a brief check-in on relevant issues that have come up since the last point of clinical contact. Then move to a review of the tracking tools that are being used to assess the individual's functioning, strengths, and challenges. Introduce potential skills that could increase stability and safety, problem solving, resiliency, and general coping. It is important to provide rationale for the skills that are being introduced. Take time to assess what the individual is already doing to cope and work collaboratively toward skill-oriented coping strategies. Define what success and failure are to the individual. Be prepared to incorporate their strengths into a clear action plan to which they are willing to commit. Introduce relevant homework and discuss any barriers to completing assignments. End the session with a review of the individual's work and their commitment to their action plan.

How do you integrate homework?

Homework is a very important tool in skills training. It is designed to generalize what is being learned and applied in session to the individual's own life. Homework is typically first addressed in the informed-consent-to-treatment phase of therapy. This is where the individual is informed about the approach and about the expectation that homework is a part of the therapeutic process. This involves discussing that one of the goals of therapy is to teach the individual skills and concepts that they can use to become more self-reliant by increasing their functioning and quality of life. Homework is then addressed in every session thereafter. There is a clear expectation that when homework is assigned, it will be created, attempted, or completed by an agreed-upon date. Therapeutic consequences for breaching the agreement need to be discussed as well. Examples might include suspending the session until the work is completed, working with the individual in session to complete the work, reassigning the homework, or updating the treatment plan to address issues with compliance. The completed homework needs then to be reviewed in each subsequent session, typically during the first part.

How do you make skills training relevant for the individual?

One of the most effective ways to make skills training relevant is to make the work experiential in session. Skills training needs to account for the individual's culture, characteristics, and preferences. The more the individual is engaged in a "hands-on" approach, the more effective the work tends to be. Practice mindfulness techniques in sessions. Incorporate stress-management techniques, such as breathing exercises, guided imagery, and progressive muscle-relaxation training. Roleplay situations and skill use to build a sense of competency with the new material being introduced. When the process of skills training is action-oriented, the individual tends to be less resistant to the process of advocating for their own change.

Teaching skills (T)

This session is not designed to be skills training. Instead, it orients the clinician to skills training in individual or group sessions.

Applying skills and concepts (A)

- Review the material for clinical integration
- Prepare experiential work involving the proposed skills and concepts
- Orient individuals to session structure and expectations
- Discuss the role of homework in the therapeutic process

Generalizing skills and concepts (G)

- Assign the individual the task of reviewing a homework sample
- Practice the process of completing homework and reviewing in session
- Problem-solve barriers to this process

General Curriculum

Notes to clinicians and individuals

- Skills training needs to be active, experiential, and relevant. The more engaged in the process is the clinician, the less resistant will be the individual.
- Be cautious about over-reliance on handouts, homework, and paper tools. Skills training is a dynamic and often quite organic process. We are creating a growth environment, not one that is sterile and impersonal.
- It takes time to become proficient with many of the skills in this manual. Many individuals find it helpful for the clinician to learn some of the skills and concepts *with* them. Be aware of your level of comfort and openness.
- It is important to remember that some skill sets are designed for movement, while others are designed to promote safety, stability, and resiliency.
- There is no right way of combining skills when introducing them. It is helpful to combine skill sets that address different aspects of functioning and needs.
- Skills tend to work most effectively when presented as combinations, as opposed to individually. There are times when it is right to focus on one skill in order to promote learning, initial use, competency, or mastery, but combining skills is the most common approach.

Session focus: Interventions and strategies

TAG
Teach – Apply – Generalize

- The goal of this session is to:
  - orient the clinician to therapeutic interventions and strategies
- Validation
- Teaching stories
- Extending
- Paradoxical interventions
- Dialectical assessment
- Context
- Psychoeducation

Interventions and strategies

Introduction of the topic
Many clinicians have training in more than one orientation to therapy. The strategies and concepts listed in this chapter are not exhaustive in scope, nor are they solely from a CBT approach. These interventions and strategies can be applied in most every session by newer clinicians to the field as well as by seasoned clinicians, for whom this section may serve as a review or as a reminder to be active and creative in therapy.

Validation
Validation may be defined as the process of establishing the soundness, accuracy, or legitimacy of something. In therapy, we often use validation to establish trust, connect with the individual, and build the therapeutic alliance. Validation takes many forms in therapy and through the course of treatment. Validation is actively listening to the individual and reflecting back to them how what they are saying has value. This value can be found in context: what the individual is experiencing makes sense given their current circumstances. It can also be found through historical reference: what the individual is experiencing makes sense given their history. Another way value can be established is through social context: what the individual is saying makes sense as most other individuals would respond in a similar manner. Validation can also take the form of sitting with the individual as a willing participant in their journey through life. This can be referred to as "proximal validation."

According to Marsha Linehan (1997), there are multiple levels of validation:

- Be awake and listen with awareness
- Reflect client's communication
- Articulate what is expressed nonverbally
- Describe how client's experience makes sense given history
- Describe how client's experience makes sense in the present context
- Be genuine

Validation is a key concept when skills training is one of the primary approaches of therapy. Skills training needs to be balanced with validation in order to actively engage the individual. Think of validation and change-oriented skills training as being on opposite ends of a continuum. Effective skills training reflects a balance between validation and teaching. There are times where validation needs to be the focus of intervention, and the same is true of skills training.

Teaching stories

A common approach to skills training is sharing stories that reflect learning opportunities. Such stories typically involve situations that represent some form of challenge to an individual, how they have responded in an ineffective manner historically, how they applied a skill set, and how they met their needs in an effective manner.

Once a relevant story demonstrating effective skill use has been shared, the process becomes a skill-training opportunity. The first step is setting the stage. This is where the details of a situation, individual, or specific predisposition are identified. The next step is to introduce a challenge that the individual struggled with, or one which they coped with in a highly effective manner. Typical coping strategies that have led to predictable results can then be identified. Problem solving additional coping skills and strategies is done while addressing anticipated outcomes of each skill or strategy. Then the individual identifies how they relate to specific or general aspects of the story and what they learned in the process. Next, they create a skills-oriented action plan, which they commit to implement. The last step is to assign the action plan as homework to be reviewed in the next session.

Extending

Extending is a process whereby the therapist actively works with an individual who is presenting with fear and/or resistance to skills-based suggestions. In a situation in which an individual is finding reasons and rationales for why any and all suggestions will not work, there is often tension: the individual feels misunderstood or pressured by the therapist, and the therapist may feel frustrated that their suggestions are being rejected out of hand. Extending provides an avenue in which to work through this process, by keeping the focus for change on the individual while externalizing the perceived rejection. This can best be explained through an example:

Chris has been in therapy to deal with health concerns and depression for a few sessions. While there is a healthy therapeutic relationship, she vacillates between attitudes of being willing to work in therapy and feeling nothing will work and that she is powerless in her own life. She struggles with being assertive with providers. The current suggestion is to attempt to use a skill set referred to as "DEAR MAN" (see the session on Adherence to Treatment Protocols), which is designed to promote healthy assertive behaviors.

Therapist (T)   Chris, we have reviewed the skill set of DEAR MAN. I am wondering, if you were to attempt to use that skill with your doctor, if you might feel like you were advocating for yourself and starting to find your voice in your appointments.

Chris (C)   That won't work. I've tried that skill before and my doctors still don't take me seriously. I just fail at everything I do!

T	That's a pretty harsh judgment you just placed on yourself.
C	I could validate that I'm trying, but what's the point? That skill doesn't help me either.
T	Is there a skill or plan that you could engage in that you would find helpful?
C	No. Nothing works for me.[1]
T	Chris, are you willing to try something new right here in session with me?
C	I'm sure whatever you have planned won't work for me. What do you want me to do?
T	I'm going to come up with a skill that you have reported effective use of in the past and then I'm going to find a reason it couldn't possibly work for you now.[2]
C	That sounds accurate for how I am feeling now. What do you want me to do?
T	Just wait and listen first. Let's go back to the skill set of DEAR MAN. If you were to use this skill, you would have a higher probability of being heard by your doctor, but even though you know the skill, there is no way he will listen. You probably won't use the skill right and he will laugh at you for trying. Does that sound accurate to where you are at right now?[3]
C	Pretty damn close!
T	I want you to identify how that skill could *accidentally* be effective.[4]
C	It would at least let him know what my needs are and what I am afraid is happening.
T	Let's reject another skill that couldn't possibly work. Validating yourself won't help because you are not even worth the effort of trying. How could that skill *accidentally* work?
C	It could accidentally help me be compassionate toward myself and give me credit for at least trying.
T	I could see where that is unacceptable and not worth trying. Let's reject another one![5]
C	[Interrupting] Wait a second, let's go back to DEAR MAN. I think I can work that skill more effectively.
T	Probably not. What's another skill that won't work?[6]
C	Is that what I've been doing? I had no idea! I can use DEAR MAN. It's worked before.

---

1 She is presenting with a clear pattern that whatever the therapist suggests will not work. If the therapist were to address this directly, she might reject this observation as well.

2 The therapist is modeling the rejecting behavior, which externalizes it from Chris as the rejection is extended to all proposed suggestions.

3 Make sure that the rejection is based in the client's experience.

4 Introduce a potentially effective alternative process.

5 Introduce irreverence to create a startling effect.

6 Stay with the extension process until the client presents with a significant shift.

T   You could try it, but that's not a clear commitment.[7]
C   I will use it in my next appointment. Can we practice it here so I'm
           ready?

Paradoxical interventions

Paradoxical interventions involve the clinician making observations about the individual's ineffective process of meeting their needs in a healthy and consistent manner. A paradox is a statement or process that seems to contradict itself, but may also be true. This indicates that logic is a core challenge to the process. If you challenge an individual with logic, the implied message is that they do not know what they are doing. This forces the individual to defend their beliefs or actions, which can lead to a power struggle in therapy. An example would be an individual who fears rejection so pushes others away with anger. As a byproduct, they feel isolated and resent others for not being close to them. Logically, this process does not make sense. If you were to challenge the behaviors with logic, there is a high probability that the individual would defend what they were doing instead of openly exploring other options. Enter the paradox and observe the process. Identify the actions and anticipated outcomes. Make observations that the intended consequences do not actually match what the individual is experiencing. Then alternatives can be explored.

Dialectical assessment

Dialectical assessment is an intervention designed to ground the individual in their own experience. It starts with the identification of a thought, behavior, emotion, or other target of treatment and places it on a continuum between opposing poles. The individual is asked to identify whether their experience is closer to one end of the continuum or the other, and by what degree. Once the individual has identified where on the continuum their experience is, that experience can be explored in relation to the distance of each of the opposing poles. An example might be an individual experiencing an urge to stop a medication. The urge is placed on a continuum between always having the urge on one end, and never having it on the other. This promotes insight into the strength of the urge in relation to its proximity to either extreme. Further assessment or exploration is then conducted in order to address probabilities of actions and potential consequences. Skill-based interventions are introduced to promote effective action plans, ending with a clear commitment for action. Dialectical assessment can be carried out with most any issue that is presented in treatment. It tends to be an effective intervention with impulsive urges, extremes in thoughts or behaviors, and when individuals lack insight into their own experience.

Context

Many individuals feel isolated and alone in their experiences. They are faced with many fears and stigmas when discussing themselves. Statements such as, "How would you know, if you've never been depressed?" and "You have no idea what I am going through!" can be quite challenging for clinicians as they attempt to connect. It is

7 Gain a clear commitment to a skills-based action plan.

imperative to provide a safe and judgment-free environment in which individuals can identify and explore their experience. Providing context can be an effective strategy with individuals who struggle to connect or express themselves. It involves the therapist using past, present, and future to align with the individual. A past-oriented context seeks to establish the "root" of the individual's experience: "Given your history, I can understand why you…" A present-oriented context seeks to focus on their current reality: "Most people would experience things similar to what you are given what is currently happening in your life." This example statement challenges the individual to entertain the possibility that they are not so unique in their current experience that it is impossible to relate. A future-oriented context looks to identify projections that the individual is having when anticipating the future: "I would be fearful of the past repeating itself, too, after going through what you have." This statement looks to name an individual's experience, while validating their struggles. There are many ways to incorporate context in therapy. Take time to connect with the client's experience, while providing a framework of understanding. This challenges the fears and stigmas that many individuals present with.

Psychoeducation
One of the key methods of engaging the individual in their treatment is by actively addressing the needs of their support system. This can be done through psychoeducation. Schedule times in therapy to invite family members and other supports to attend. Provide information to these supports about therapy, its tools, and its process. One suggested method is to host a family/support member session that meets once monthly for 1.5 hours. The first 45 minutes are dedicated to presenting skills-based materials and teaching some of the skills and concepts that are routinely used in therapy. This provides information and starts to bridge toward a common language. Many support members do not know how to help or what to say. Skills provide a common language that can instill understanding and hope. The last 45 minutes are typically dedicated to Q&;A with the therapist(s). This is important time in which supports can address any needs and concerns that they may have. Informed supports are key to healthy growth and action for the individual in therapy.

Notes to clinicians and individuals

- Validation is not agreeing with the individual, it is connecting with their experience. This skill takes practice! One of the main goals is to model this in session so the individual can learn self-validation.
- Stories are a great way to connect. They promote understanding, skill development, and connection, and can challenge unhealthy beliefs.
- Extending is an advanced therapeutic strategy. Practice with your peers to gain proficiency. It can be a very powerful intervention, but needs a strong therapeutic alliance.
- When engaging in extending interventions, you may need to externalize the example from the individual to get distance from their immediate experience. When they can see their own process from a new perspective separate from themselves, they tend to be more open to discussing their patterns and the impact they have

on their functioning. If you directly challenge them, they may withdraw and become defensive, as though you are pushing them too hard or minimizing their experience.

- Dialectical assessment can become a fun intervention for all. I routinely dedicate time in therapy to playing "stump the therapist," where individuals challenge me to place their examples on a continuum. This is typically done monthly, at their request.
- Psychoeducation is extremely important. Individuals reference our work with their support systems as some of the most important we do. They identify their supports as having common skills to reference, being appropriately supportive and challenging, and being engaged with them in their treatment and their lives.

Session focus: Safety assessment and contracting

TAG
Teach – Apply – Generalize

- The goal of this session is to:
  - Discuss the need for safety assessment and contracting for safety
  - Provide a suggested course of action for addressing safety concerns
  - Provide an example of a safety assessment
  - Provide an example of a safety contract
- What to discuss:
  - Safety policies and protocols
  - Safety and self-injury
  - Relevant forms
- Skills to teach:
  - This is an assessment and contracting session
- Generalize:
  - Create an action plan for a **Safety Contract** (see handout)
  - Create an action plan for a **Skills Implementation Plan** (see handout)
  - Problem-solve barriers
  - Commit to the individual's plan
  - Review in every session
- Review goal sheet

Safety assessment and contracting

Introduction of the topic
Many clinicians have little or no training in safety assessment. Graduate schools may address the topic, but typically in some generic or sterile manner. Most training happens when the clinician is practicing in the field. It is not a question of *if* you will encounter an individual who is suicidal, but *when* you will encounter an individual who is suicidal. Individuals with a diagnosis of cancer have a completion rate of more than twice the national average. Safety is a true concern, and something to be taken seriously at all times. A thorough assessment and potential safety contracting provide the clinician invaluable information to assist in making decisions. When safety is a primary issue in therapy, it can be unnerving for the clinician, which further highlights the need for a clear direction in a time of crisis. This can be achieved through training and by adopting protocols, which you should inform all clients about at the start of therapy through informed consent to treatment.

Policy and procedure
Most every agency has policies and procedures that serve as a guide for handling many common events. Content typically ranges from what to do in case of a tornado all the way to the agency's hiring/firing procedures. It is common practice to sign an

employment agreement that indicates that within the first week, the policy and procedure manual will be reviewed. Manuals may or may not address what to do with a suicidal individual. The recommended first step is to have a thorough understanding of what the agency considers to be best practice when this event occurs. It is my strongest suggestion that a set of policies and procedures be created to address this issue if it is not already in place.

Here are a list of areas to consider when reviewing safety policies and procedures:

- **Informed consent** – Do all individuals know your policies and procedures pertaining to safety?
- **Assessment protocol** – What is the procedure and what safety tools are used in the process?
- **Safety contracting** – When is this appropriate, and what tools are used in the process?
- **Transporting** – If individuals are deemed high-risk, when and how are they transported to a higher LOC?
- **Documentation** – What is documented, and when?
- **Consultation** – When does consultation occur, and what are the limits on autonomy in making decisions on behalf of the high-risk individual?
- **Training** – Does training on safety occur upon employment and periodically thereafter?
- **Supervision** – Is there adequate supervision of the clinician and the individual?
- **Restraint** – Is restraint used in any manner and is the individual ever left alone?

Assessment versus therapy

Assessment and therapy both have a role in treatment. High-risk individuals present a unique challenge at times in therapy, forcing the clinician to balance their treatment strategies. Assessment provides crucial information about the current state of the individual, while therapy can be considered an ongoing and dynamic process. When safety is in question, assessment may be the most effective course of action. Adopting the stance of assessment has a completely different feel and tone. It is very matter-of-fact, directive, and may involve forced choice on behalf of the individual. Attempting to conduct therapy with a suicidal individual can lead to confusion and the individual not receiving the help that they truly need.

Assessment is a process of suspending a therapeutic work while attempting to gather information about the current state of the individual. It is an information-gathering technique that targets risk factors for the individual. It typically involves a series of closed-ended questions led by the clinician that solicit "yes or no" responses or short answers. Therapy is a process involving open-ended questions targeting self-exploration. There are many forms of therapy, and many corresponding styles. The major difference between assessment and therapy (regarding safety) is that the process of assessment is brief and highly directive. Although it relies on the therapeutic alliance, assessment may lead the clinician to act on behalf of the individual in an attempt to keep them safe.

Here are some guidelines to consider when adopting the stance of assessment:

- Orient clients to your safety procedures: if x, then y. Use clear contingencies.
- Use consistent follow-through
- Take all suicidal comments seriously: there are no "games"
- Safety is a "yes" or "no," with a clear safety plan
- Safety assessment and planning happen in the time allotted
- Negotiations stop at the end of the session

Safety assessment

There are many versions of safety assessments. Some clinicians gather data through forms and direct questioning, while others rely on direct questions only. Here is a list of questions and reminders I suggest you consider.

- Ideation or urges present? Assess level
- Plan present?
- Intent present?
- Method?
- Access?
- Lethality?
- History?
- Consider additional risk factors
- Assessment is matter of fact
- Communicate and consult
- Document fully at the time of service

Case example

This example is intended to demonstrate the point about taking all discussions concerning safety seriously.

Bob is a 34-year-old male with a history of depression. He was diagnosed with prostate cancer 8 months before being referred for therapy. He presents with average intelligence, a willingness to work in therapy, and a high degree of demoralization, as his bills are pushing his financial resources and his physical health has begun to deteriorate. The therapist has worked with Bob for a few sessions and is starting to develop a trusting therapeutic relationship. Bob has just identified that "It would be easier on me and my family if I weren't such a burden anymore." The therapist quickly moves from a therapeutic exploration-based stance to one of assessment.

THERAPIST (T)   Bob, can you clarify your last statement please?
BOB (B)   Sure, life would be easier if I weren't around anymore. I've been thinking about just ending it all. I'm done with the pain and what I am putting my family through.
T   Bob, are you currently experiencing suicidal thoughts?
B   I don't know, maybe.
T   It needs to be a yes or no answer. Are you currently experiencing suicidal thoughts?
B   Yes. I would never hurt anyone else. I'm the problem.
T   Are the thoughts low, moderate, or highly intrusive?
B   High.

T	Do you intend to act on these urges or ideas?
B	I think so, yes.
T	Do you have a plan of killing yourself?
B	Yes.
T	What is the method?
B	Overdosing. I would mix pills and alcohol.
T	Do you have access to the pills and alcohol?
B	They are at my house. Please don't tell my family! This would crush them!
T	Would this plan potentially be lethal?
B	Yes, I researched the combination on the Internet. It would work for sure. If not, I would find something for sure.
T	Do you have any history acting on urges like this in the past?
B	No. I never have. I have never felt this way before, either.

Bob clearly gives answers that are alarming and that require the therapist to act in good faith to address his safety concerns. The encounter ends with Bob agreeing to call 911 from the therapist's office. Together, they inform emergency responders of Bob's willingness to participate in the assessment process, as well as his willingness to be assessed further at the hospital. They identify his current risk for safety and the need for assessment for admittance. The therapist makes a copy of Bob's identifying information sheet from his chart for Bob, the emergency responders, and the hospital. Bob is open and honest with the emergency responders when they arrive. While he is being transported, the therapist places calls to the hospital to assist in their assessment process and to his entire treatment team to update them on Bob's status.

This will be addressed further in the "Notes to Clinicians and Individuals" section.

Safety contracts and skills implementation plans

A **Safety Contract** can be an important tool when addressing safety concerns with individuals. It is important to create one before it is needed. I typically have all clients complete a safety contract and a skills implementation plan within the first few weeks of therapy. It is better for clients to have access to tools that they participated in creating before a time of crisis. This represents an approach designed to be proactive instead of reactive in therapy.

Safety contracts are truly valued through the depth of the therapeutic alliance. They are not about defense strategies in a court of law: they are a therapeutic tool to assist individuals in the process of contracting for safety. When an individual is experiencing suicidal thoughts or urges, but demonstrates the willingness and ability to maintain safety, safety contracts can be useful in ensuring they do. They commonly take the form of a promise or agreement that the individual will honor their commitment to stay safe by following a predetermined safety plan. Such plans involve skills work, connecting to support systems, and using appropriate non-emergency services to maintain safety. Safety contracts must incorporate emergency services if the individual becomes unsafe at any time.

A **Skills Implementation Plan** is a therapeutic tool that rates distress from low to high and promotes skill use at every level. It identifies bands of distress from 0–2 (low) to 9–10 (crisis). It incorporates skills that can be used at each assessment level and indentifies the resources available to promote healthy coping. Associated thoughts, feelings, and behaviors are identified to promote insight into where the individual is currently functioning and how they can (i) not make the situation worse and (ii) increase their functioning and/or quality of life.

Teaching skills (T)

This session is not designed to be skills training. It outlines the need and proposed plan and process for addressing safety issues.

Applying skills and concepts (A)

- Create an action plan for a **Safety Contract**
- Create an action plan for a **Skills Implementation Plan**
- Problem-solve barriers to this process

Generalizing skills and concepts (G)

- Assign individuals the task of completing their safety contracts and skills implementation plans at the start of therapy
- Assign individuals the task of reviewing their work with their support system and treatment team

Notes to clinicians and individuals

- Stay calm. When an individual presents with safety concerns, it can be very intense and intimidating. Seek support and get other clinicians involved at the earliest stage possible. Never leave a suicidal individual alone!
- Assessment and risk-management needs to be the focus of the interaction. Get information. If the individual is not responding clearly or following the line of questioning, you may have to engage in forced-choice Q&A: "If you do not correct me, then I will assume that the answer is yes [or no, depending on the question being asked]."
- Ethics codes promote autonomy on behalf of the individual seeking treatment. Every clinician needs to review their code of ethics and understand the implications of acting on behalf of "high-risk" individuals.
- Make sure to have confidentiality releases for all team members, including emergency providers, signed at the start of therapy.
- Care coordination is crucial during a crisis. Let all team members know what is happening and what the plan is regarding safety.
- All transports are through emergency services or 911. This limits the risk of the individual acting impulsively when leaving your care. If the individual called by phone, stay connected and coach them to the nearest emergency facility.
- Imbed the individual in the entire process, if appropriate. If you fear that they will elope (run), you may have to alter your process accordingly.

- Documentation is always at the time of service. This is considered "best practice" and will also reduce potential liability.
- Consulting other professionals on safety and other clinical matters is a strength, not a weakness for clinicians. If you find yourself questioning what to do, consult, and always err on the side of safety!
- Get training and supervision on this topic if is an area of growth for you. Few clinicians feel well trained in the area of safety.
- When contracting for safety, you are extending the individual's commitment to the next professional contact.
- The safety contract handout is generic and may need to be modified to fit your practice.

Session focus: Cognitive and behavioral analysis

TAG
Teach – Apply – Generalize

- The goal of this session is to:
  - Orient the clinician to cognitive analysis
  - Orient the clinician to behavioral analysis
- What to discuss:
  - Pattern recognition
  - Increasing insight
  - Relevant forms:
    - **Cognitive Mapping** (see handout)
    - **Behavioral Mapping** (see handout)
- Skills to teach:
  - Problem solving
  - Observe, Describe, Participate
- Generalize:
  - Create an action plan to complete a cognitive analysis
  - Create an action plan to complete a behavioral analysis
  - Problem-solve barriers
  - Commit to the individual's plan
  - Review in the next session

Cognitive and behavioral analysis

Introduction of the topic

Many individuals struggle with recognizing their patterns of thinking and behaving. When an individual is experiencing a chronic illness such as cancer, there is a lot of doubt, fear, chaos, and unpredictability. When faced with such significant challenges to wellness and functioning, it is common for individuals to revert back to old patterns of thinking and behaving that have worked for them in the past. These old patterns have historically met needs in some way. As a result, they have been reinforced and tend to be repeated in many areas of their lives. When faced with the new and distinctive challenges that cancer often presents, these patterns may not be effective in meeting the individual's needs and may not generalize well to many areas of their functioning. The patterns may be applied in a way that is ineffective, sporadic, and lacking in purposeful direction. The aims of introducing behavioral and cognitive analyses are to promote insight and pattern recognition. When an individual can increase their ability to understand what they are doing, when they are attempting to intervene, and why they are engaging in a process, they have an opportunity to be more skillful. This increase in skill can promote an increase in functioning and quality of life that increases the probability of meeting their needs in a more effective manner. There are three major benefits to the individual:

- **Remoralization** – The process of increasing one's ability to challenge feelings of demoralization while increasing overall resiliency
- **Increased insight into their own functioning** – Increasing the individual's ability and motivation to meet their needs in a healthy manner
- **Increased ability to be proactive instead of being reactive** – Reorienting the individual toward action as opposed to reaction

Cognitive analysis

The goals of conducting a cognitive analysis are to increase motivation (remoralization), increase insight, and increase effectiveness through a process of exploration. This tool can be used when individuals are struggling with a situation or when they have made progress in an area and it would be helpful to explore their experience further. The clinician is encouraged to identify when the individual is using a skill or skills effectively, or when a skill could have been used to promote a more effective approach. See the **Cognitive Mapping** handout.

Orientation

This is the starting point of the analysis. It provides the individual's view of the world, through three main lenses: attitude, beliefs, and expectations. Attitudes may be defined as an individual's expression of favor or disfavor toward a person, place, thing, or event. This is important to explore, as it ranges from positive outlooks and evaluations to negative ones. Ambivalence is also important for some individuals, as it may represent an indicator of demoralization and lack of participation in one's own life. Beliefs may be defined as an individual's mental representation of the likelihood of truth. What someone believes to be true, or what they believe likely to be true, drives both thought and behavioral probabilities. Expectations may be defined as what an individual expects to happen, or believes will happen based on their actions and inactions. This is a very important aspect to explore, since individuals have a higher probability of acting in a manner that is consistent with their expectations. If an individual expects a positive outcome, they tend to act in a positive manner. If an individual expects a negative outcome, they tend to lead with inaction or ambivalence.

Event

The second step in the analysis is when an event occurs that captures the individual's attention for some reason. This event could be either internal (a thought or feeling comes to attention) or external (something happens in the individual's environment). Events occur all of the time, whether internal or external. Many are routine and require little or no attention on behalf of the individual. This step is important to explore, since it is capturing attention, which is one of the first steps in evaluation. It is common to label the event as "internal" or "external" and to note why attention was given.

Interpretation/templates

The next step is interpretation. Consider template-matching theory, where sensory information is compared to copies (templates) housed in the long-term memory (LTM). Sensory information is processed to make sense of the information with which the individual is presented. This is the individual's immediate evaluation of the event. Such a reaction tends to occur through one of the primary filters of their orientation. It begins to trigger a chain of evaluations led by their attitudes, beliefs, or expectations. Confirmation bias needs to be addressed with individuals experiencing chronic illness. Sensory information may lead such an individual to pay attention only to information that validates their fears, while missing information that suggests they are misplaced. This is a primary starting point for skillful interventions. The clinician is encouraged to explore the immediate interpretation and how it either meets needs or presents as a barrier to effective functioning. It is also important to explore the other orientations, since this may lead to a higher degree of balance and may present the individual with more information and options to explore.

Schemas

The next step in the analysis incorporates concepts of pattern recognition. The event and the immediate interpretation are typically compared to previous experiences, to provide context, meaning, and further processing. Once the individual is able to begin to make sense of the information, they organize the experience through schemas. A schema is a structured pattern of behavior or thought that organizes categories of information. Schemas also organize relationships between and among actions and thoughts. Individuals use schemas to organize current knowledge and provide a framework for future understanding. This step represents the process of pattern recognition and ascribing meaning. It is crucial to explore, since the processing at this level tends to be more in-depth.

Reality (hypothesis) checking

The next step is to check whether the individual's interpretation or experience matches the facts that are available. It is quite common for individuals to interpret information through fear of what is or might be happening, and not to check to see if their fears are founded. It is important to gather as many facts as are available and to create a hypothesis that can be either proven or disproven. This step slows the process down and encourages the individual to check their experience against the facts. It also assists in the creation of a belief that can be verified. The individual needs to incorporate others into this process as well (e.g., medical doctors, nurses, Internet searches, peers, members of their support system). This challenges isolation and inaction, through the inclusion of others.

Action planning

The next step is to create an action plan to test the belief. This involves gathering data, brainstorming testing ideas, and problem solving any barriers to the process. It is important to create a clear plan that involves other individuals and to establish timelines in which to complete this step.

Anticipated consequences

Once an action plan has been created, anticipated consequences need to be explored. This step represents a wide range of options and possibilities. It may be important to define what "success" and "failure" mean to the individual. If the goal of testing the belief is to challenge their thinking, behaviors, or feelings, the individual may be presented with painful or positive information.

Re-evaluation of the plan

Once all of the available information has been gathered, a plan has been created, and the potential consequences have been identified, it is important to spend some time reviewing the plan and getting a firm commitment from the individual for follow-through. Motivation is often a primary challenge for individuals experiencing a chronic illness such as cancer. Taking time to gather resources and lead with the individual's strengths can be key to compliance.

Action

This incorporates both thoughts and behaviors. It is important to identify which thoughts are paired with which behaviors. This is a key step in the pattern-recognition process.

Consequences/outcomes

This is an analysis of the consequences and outcomes of the action step. The results need to be viewed through the lenses of the real and the perceived: there may be discrepancies between what is believed to have happened and what actually occurred. This last step either confirms or challenges the individual's orientation to the world.

Behavioral analysis

The goals of conducting a behavioral analysis are to increase motivation (remoralization), increase insight, and increase effectiveness through a process of exploration. The core concept is to select a behavior that you want to analyze for effectiveness by identifying what happened before it was adopted and what happened after. A behavioral analysis is a therapeutic tool. It can be used when individuals are struggling with a situation or when they have made progress in an area and it would be helpful to explore their experience further. The clinician is encouraged to identify when the individual is using a skill or skills effectively, or when a skill could have been used to promote more effective action(s).

In the **Behavioral Mapping** handout, the analysis starts with predisposition and follows a timeline (the arrow in the background) through consequences. Each box represents a stage, phase, or progression in the process. The arrow may represent the movement of time, an overall process, or the rising intensity toward BA. The smaller arrows represent movement or progression between boxes. Please note that movement can be either progression or regression, which accounts for the possibility of an individual cycling between aspects of the model. This is important, since individuals may progress through the model in a stepwise and sequential manner, or they may cycle between aspects as if they were phases and not stages. This flexibility is designed to account for the complexity of movement through and within the model of functioning. The triangle above the "Integrated Response" box represents the psychological complexity of integrating thoughts, feelings, and behaviors when the individual begins the process of incorporating these three main aspects of functioning.

Predisposition

This is the starting point of the analysis. There are two main factors to consider when exploring behaviors at this point: action and vulnerability. It is important to identify whether the individual is prone to action or inaction, and for what reasons. Demoralization from chronic conditions can set the stage for an individual's energy levels, as well as their tendency to act and react in certain ways. Vulnerability is another important factor to assess. What might make the individual vulnerable to the prompting event? Lack of sleep, pain, inconsistent self-cares, ambivalence, and being emotionally charged by fear or anxiety are just a few areas to consider when exploring vulnerability.

Event

The second step or phase in the analysis is when an event occurs that captures the individual's attention for some reason. This event might be either internal (a thought or a feeling comes to attention) or external (something happens in the individual's environment). Events occur all of the time, whether internal or external. Many are routine and require little to no attention on behalf of the individual. This step is important to explore, since it is capturing attention, which is one of the first steps in evaluation. It is common to label the event as "internal" or "external" and to note why attention was given.

Interpretation

The next step or phase is when the individual interprets the event. Consider template-matching theory, where the incoming sensory information is compared directly to copies (templates) stored in the LTM. These copies are stored in the process of our past experiences and learning. Sensory information is processed to make sense of the information with which the individual is presented. This is the individual's immediate evaluation of the event. Such a reaction tends to occur through one of the primary filters of their orientation. It begins to trigger a chain of evaluations led by their attitudes, beliefs, or expectations. Confirmation bias needs to be addressed with individuals experiencing chronic illness. Sensory information may lead such an individual to pay attention only to information that validates their fears, while missing information that suggests they are misplaced. This is a primary starting point for skillful interventions. The clinician is encouraged to explore the immediate interpretation and how it either meets needs or presents as a barrier to effective functioning. It is also important to explore the other orientations, since this may lead to a higher degree of balance and may present the individual with more information and options to explore.

Physiological response

The next step or phase is the body's "hardwired" response to the situation. This is the first behavioral response to note, and it includes fight, flight, or freeze. Primary emotional responses of fear, anger, joy, and grief may also be present. The main consideration is to identify how the individual is responding physiologically. Creating a list can often be helpful for pattern recognition. For example, a racing heart, flushed face, or trembling body may be an indicator of a stress response, which can trigger a behavioral reaction of fight (defense against a perceived threat), flight (a flee response from a perceived threat), or freeze (an inactive behavioral response designed to neutralize oneself as a target from a perceived threat).

Integrated response

The next step or phase incorporates a very complex integration for the individual, involving thoughts, feelings, and behaviors. When taking a balanced/planful approach, this is where the individual can purposefully gather as much information as possible from a multitude of sources and prepare for action. One modality of functioning tends to be primary at this time, if the individual is out of balance. If thinking is the primary modality of functioning, the individual's focus is on their internal process (schemas, anticipated outcomes, self-talk), which may prepare them for action. If behavior is the primary modality, there are two main responses to explore. Planful behaviors incorporate data from all three modalities, with a movement toward problem solving as preparation for action. Reactive behaviors tend to minimize, expand, or distort information, which leads to escape, avoidance, or alteration of functioning in some manner. If emotion (primary/secondary/tertiary) is the primary modality of functioning, this can lead to impulsive behaviors. Impulsivity is behavior without adequate thought, the tendency to act with less forethought than most individuals of equal ability and knowledge, or a predisposition toward rapid, unplanned reactions to internal or external stimuli, without regard to the negative consequences of these reactions (www.impulsivity.org).

Action

This is the behavior that is being targeted for analysis. The overall goal of the analysis is to target behaviors either to keep and reinforce or to modify in order to meet needs in a healthier manner.

Consequences

The last step or phase in the analysis is to identify the consequences of the behavior. Identify the consequences for others as well as for the individual. A behavior may be very effective in meeting a need for an individual but alienate them from their support system. A common example of this is an anger response to criticism. The anger response makes the individual feel less vulnerable by pushing others away, but it may lead to isolation if used too much. It is also important to identify consequences that are real (verifiable by others) versus perceived (known only to the individual). This can potentially identify attribution errors, which are a common form of distortion and a strong motivator for behavior.

Teaching skill

- **Observe** – Noticing one's experience.
- **Describe** – The process of putting words on one's experience.
- **Participate** – What the individual is doing to cope with the current situation and how present they are in the process.

Notes to clinicians and individuals

- Skills-based interventions and general therapeutic interventions can be conducted at any step in either of the models, or between different steps.
- Be cautious of overuse of these forms and processes. If they are relied upon too often, they can lose meaning, and even be viewed as a punishment.
- A cognitive analysis can be performed when an individual is struggling with a situation, in order to promote insight through pattern recognition. It can also be conducted when they are functioning effectively, in order to promote a strength-based approach.
- The clinician is encouraged to be creative with these tools and to adapt them to the individual seeking services.
- Two forms of analysis are presented. Thus, the clinician has the option to use either a thorough approach (integration of both cognitive and behavioral) or a more simplified and straightforward one (use of either alone).
- Note that these processes are cyclical in nature. Individuals can progress through the cycle and can get stuck between steps. This accounts for the possibility that individuals may progress through either model with one aspect of functioning while being quite stuck with another.
- It is common for individuals not to want to engage in this process. Insight is challenging, and working toward change is hard, tedious, and can take a lot of effort. A common reaction to distress is to escape, avoid, or alter responses in an attempt to cope. Analyzing these reactions is quite challenging.
- Processing either analysis is extremely important in advocating for healthier functioning. Discuss why the analysis is being suggested, the potential benefits that can be gained, and the need to obtain a clear commitment to practice what is learned when completing the process.
- An additional goal of analysis is to slow the process, bring to light the steps/stages/phases involved, and integrate skillful interventions throughout.

Session focus: Self-regulation and illness perceptions

TAG
Teach – Apply – Generalize

- The goal of this session is to:
  - Discuss the role of self-regulation in health behavior
  - Increase the individual's understanding of their perceptions of their illness
  - Assess the individual using the Illness Perception Questionnaire – Revised (IPQ-R) (Moss-Morris et al., 2002)
  - Increase treatment compliance
- What to discuss:
  - Self-regulation
  - Identity
  - Cause
  - Timeline
  - Consequences
  - Cure/control
  - Illness coherence
  - Control versus influence
- Skills to teach:
  - Assessment of the individual using the IPQ-R
- Generalize:
  - Create an action plan to engage the individual in the process of **Goal Setting** (see handout)
  - Problem-solve barriers
  - Commit to the individual's plan
  - Review in the next session
- Review goal sheet

Self-regulation and illness perceptions

Introduction of the topic

This session is designed to orient the clinician to self-regulation and illness perceptions, in order to promote increased compliance and functioning for individuals seeking treatment.

Self-regulation is the process of goal setting and goal striving, and includes dealing with a range of challenges that individuals may face when trying to achieve something that is important but, almost by definition, difficult to attain (Mischel et al., 1996). The term "self-regulation" is often used to refer broadly to efforts by humans to alter their thoughts, feelings, desires, and actions in the perspective of such higher goals (Carver & Scheier, 1998). Consider self-regulation as a dynamic process of setting goals, developing and implementing strategies in order to achieve the goals, evaluating the process, and revising the goals and strategies when needed. Managing emotional responses and altering cognitive processes can lead to greater efficacy in goal attainment. The probability of goal attainment increases when the goal is considered to be personally meaningful, when the individual anticipates positive outcomes, and when they have the ability to influence the process. This encourages the individual to be an active participant in their own treatment. Successful self-regulation involves the effective management of a self-directed change process, with potentially competing goals across the course of time. This indicates that there may be times when short-term and long-term goals are actually conflictual. Efficacy requires the individual to be their own agent of change and to prioritize their wants and needs in a changing environment. One of the most challenging self-regulatory tasks is maintaining tenacity in goal pursuit in the face of difficult or frustrating situations (Mischel et al., 1996). Distractions and temptations are often regarded as the main causes of self-regulatory failure (Baumeister & Heatherton, 1996).

Self-regulation models and theories apply well to behavioral health. The focus is on the individual who is active and directive in their own treatment process. It encourages the individual to set realistic goals, engage in active problem solving, and evaluate their current care plans, while managing emotions and challenging ineffective cognitions. The approach provides little information on the role of coping in staying on track during goal pursuit and treatment compliance. This is where skill training can bridge the gap between short-term and long-term goal attainment, as well as improving treatment compliance. In order to accomplish this task effectively, the individual's illness perceptions need to be assessed and integrated into the goal-setting and attainment process.

Illness perceptions

Recent research indicates that a client's illness perceptions may be more predictive of treatment adherence and receptivity to treatment than other explanations (Broadbent et al., 2006). This indicates the importance of assessing and exploring an individual's illness perceptions in order to promote compliance and engagement in treatment.

According to Diefenbach (2014):

> Illness representations are patients' beliefs and expectations about an illness or somatic symptom. Illness representations are central to Leventhal's Self-Regulation Theory…[which] postulates that illness representations determine a person's appraisal of an illness situation and health behavior. The self-regulation framework is conceptualized as a parallel processing framework. One processing arm is dedicated to the cognitive process-ing of an internal or external stimulus and the second, parallel processing arm is dedicated to the processing of the emotional aspects of that stimulus. One implication of this par-allel processing is that health behaviors can be triggered as a result of cognitive as well as emotional processes (Leventhal, Diefenbach, & Leventhal, 1992).

More concretely, research has identified six attributes or components of illness repre-sentations:

- **Identity** – The name or label of a threat (e.g., sore throat, arthritis).
- **Timeline** – The threat's believed time trajectory (e.g., acute, chronic, cyclical).
- **Consequences** – The believed consequence of a threat (minor or major).

- **Cause** – The threat's causal mechanism (e.g., hereditary, external, internal).
- **Control/cure** – Whether something can be done to control the threat (Lau & Hartmann, 1983).
- **Illness coherence** – Whether a person thinks about the threat in a coherent way (Weinman et al., 1986).

The following example is intended to help explain how attributes construct an illness representation: A woman detects an unusual lump in her breast. For a lot of women, the first thought that comes to mind is "cancer" (identity). The cancer label will trigger thoughts about suffering and potentially life-threatening consequences, prolonged treatment (cure), and probably uncertain cause beliefs. Simultaneously, an intense emotional reaction of anxiety and fear will be triggered. This is the reason cancer is often times called a "hot cognition," where illness representations and their affective reactions are fused together.

Control versus influence
It is important to identify how the individual perceives control in their lives and how this perception or belief affects their functioning. "Control" may be defined as "having power over something." A common belief is that if a person views themselves as "being in control", they *should* be able to exert their power and force change. This can be very positive when the change that the person desires *can* be made reality through their efforts. A problem arises when the situation or an individual's response is resistant to being controlled. If they attempt to exert their power and do not get the desired result, they become polarized in their interpretation: "I failed," "I needed to work harder or do more." Polarized interpretations lead to all-or-nothing and black-and-white thinking. This reduces freedom of acceptable experience, restricts choices, and makes it difficult for the individual to take responsibility for their actions. This may become clearer through a common example: Many individuals believe that they can "control" their emotions. If emotions could truly be controlled, however, there would be no use for medication-management or psychotherapy: people would simply exert their power and choose not to be depressed or anxious. The belief that things can be controlled implies that there is a clear and predictable course of action that leads to one acceptable outcome. This belief does not generalize well to the reality that most individuals experience.

"Influence" may be defined as "producing some effect without exerting direct control or power." If an individual focuses their attention on exerting influence, they have more choices and possibilities. Influence challenges all-or-nothing and black-and-white thinking. This concept can be clarified by continuing the previous example: Replace the belief that emotions can be controlled with the belief that emotions can be influenced. This change implies that there is no *one* clear course of action that leads to *one* acceptable outcome. The individual does not have to be perfect in their approach to a situation, and can accept that change is a process that is at times dynamic and unpredictable. This shift allows for flexibility in beliefs, interpretations, choices, actions, and acceptable outcomes. There is now a range of what is allowable or acceptable, which can make it easier for the individual to take responsibility for their actions and their involvement in the treatment process.

Clinical integration

One of the primary treatment goals is to increase the individual's functioning and quality of life. Self-regulation is a key factor in this movement. The individual needs to take ownership of their treatment and be the leader of their treatment team. This encourages them to be active and planful in their treatment. To accomplish this task, it is important first to assess the individual's illness perceptions. This will give the clinician valuable information about their relationship with their illness and will set the stage for goal setting and treatment planning. Discuss the illness perceptions in relation to making meaning and motivation for change. Strengths and barriers will emerge through dialogue. A strength-based approach is strongly encouraged when exploring these areas with clients. Begin discussions about their vision of recovery (VOR), making sure to highlight what they are already doing effectively and what resources can assist them in the process of advocating for their own change. Challenge the perception of control and the individual's views when they emerge as a barrier. Many things in our lives are out of our control, but we do have influence in how we respond to events. This process will assist in promoting open communication, enabling discussion of strengths and perceived barriers, and orienting the individual toward ownership in the treatment process. As a potential result, self-regulation will begin to increase.

Teaching skills (T)

This session is not designed to be skills training. It outlines the concepts of self-regulation and illness perceptions for the clinician.

Applying skills and concepts (A)

- Create an action plan for completing the IPQ-R
- Problem-solve barriers to this process
- Once the IPQ-R is completed, discuss the results with the individual

Generalizing skills and concepts (G)

- Assign the individual the task of reviewing the **Goal Setting** handout and homework and prepare for the next session
- Problem-solve barriers to this process

Notes to clinicians and individuals

- The responsibility for change is always an open topic of discussion. When working with experts and specialists, it is easy for the individual to forget or minimize their role in their own treatment.
- Assessment and evaluation is a dynamic and ongoing process between the individual and their treatment team members.
- Strengths are always present, but they may be hard to identify in times of crisis. Have patience.
- It may be an important part of the change process to define success and failure. I commonly define success as any and all attempts to advocate for oneself regardless

of the outcome. Failure is then viewed as a lack of self-regulation and/or advocacy. This tends to be a primary barrier for many individuals when engaging in their treatment.

- Take your time in the initial assessment phase of therapy. Gather information and work on the therapeutic relationship. Therapy is effectively done *with* individuals, not *to* them.

Session focus: Chronic illness

TAG
Teach – Apply – Generalize

- The first goal of this session is to orient the clinician to the stages of cancer
- The second goal of this session is to orient the clinician to a phase model of chronic illness
- What to discuss:
  - Phase 1: Crisis
  - Phase 2: Stabilization
  - Phase 3: Resolution
  - Phase 4: Integration

Chronic illness

Introduction of the topic

Stages of cancer
According to the Cancer Institute NSW (2015):

> The term "stage of cancer" means the stage the cancer was at when it was first diagnosed. Being sure about the stage is very important because it is a critical factor in deciding the best way to treat the cancer.

Stage is also very important to prognosis – prediction of the cancer's effect on the person who has it. On average, the higher the stage, the worse the cancer's effect.

- **Stage 0: "In situ"** – "A cell that becomes a cancer cell usually does so in the company of other similar cells. Often, but not always, it can produce a tumour right there in that tissue, in a way that poses little or no threat to life" (Cancer Institute NSW, 2015).
- **Stage 1: Localized cancer** – "At the next stage, the cancer cells gain the ability to pass through the 'basement membrane,' that is the thin, fibrous boundary to the tissue in which the cancer began, and to invade neighbouring tissue. This invasion is a serious step, because it indicates that the growing cancer cells may threaten life" (Cancer Institute NSW, 2015).
- **Stages 2 and 3: Regional spread** – "Once a cancer cell has invaded, a common next step is for one of its daughter cells to invade through a lymph vessel…Sometimes, though, it divides and forms a lump in the lymph node. This stage is often referred to as regional spread. That is, the cancer has spread within the general region in which it first began but not to other parts of the body" (Cancer Institute NSW, 2015).
- **Stage 4: Distant spread** – "The next step can be quite varied. Cells from the lump in the lymph node may spread further through lymph vessels to more distant lymph

nodes or on into the blood stream. Or cells from the original lump may invade a capillary and enter the blood stream that way" (Cancer Institute NSW, 2015).

This section is designed to orient the clinician to the four-phase model of chronic illness developed by Patricia Fennell (2003).

It is important to understand the process of maturation and change for individuals with chronic illness. Many of us are familiar with the transtheoretical model of change. This model accounts for intentional behavioral change starting from precontemplation, moving through multiple stages, and ending with maintenance. Conceptually, individuals go through the stages in a stepwise and sequential manner. Individuals who are experiencing chronic illness often struggle to advocate for their own change; more commonly, change is forced upon them and they find themselves reacting. Since their illness is chronic in nature, a stepwise model may not account for the ongoing challenges they experience or the variability of course their illness may take. Patricia Fennell (2003) outlined a four-phase approach to viewing chronic illness, which captures its complexity and variability.

What to discuss
Cancer may not be a one-time event. It can return multiple times over the course of an individual's life, and can even become a chronic (ongoing) illness that never fully goes away.

According to Fennell (2003):

The model examines the phenomenon of chronicity and the varieties of traumatization that can be experienced by the chronically ill. The approach assumes that patients who successfully navigate the four phases will achieve *integration* rather than cure. Because of this changed goal, clinicians engage in a shift of viewpoint and undertake new activities. In addition to ensuring that their patients receive standard medical care, clinicians following this model seek to provide palliation for their patients, guide them toward strategies for dealing with their life situation, and engage with them in discussions of the philosophical or spiritual dimensions of their situation.

The new model defines four broad phases experienced by the chronically ill – crisis, stabilization, resolution, and integration. For each phase, the model describes the events and responses that typically occur in each context of the patient's life – that is, within the physical and psychological self and within the family, clinical setting, workplace, community, and culture at large – and identifies methods of assessment and treatment for that phase. Each phase also addresses the changing experiences of the clinician and provides direction so that clinicians may best incorporate these changing experiences.

The model recognizes that patients may move backward as well as forward among the phases because lapses of insight or new crises of illness or life situation may return the patient to experiences characteristic of earlier phases (Berg, Evangelista, & Dunbar-Jacob, 2002[...]). After patients and clinicians have negotiated the four phases once, however, they have learned to anticipate the experience of relapse in their illness or untoward new experience; and after the initial shock, they know better how to deal with it...Whereas they must again use the techniques of earlier phases to address new issues, the time spent moving into resolution and integration diminishes.

The Four-Phase Model...employs the term *phase* rather than *stage* because it does not regard the phases as discrete entities, and patients do not necessarily pass through them only once. Phases can, in fact, recur and may overlap, resulting in more than one phase occurring concurrently ([...]Kübler-Ross, 1969).

Sperry modifies this model and presents it as follows.

Phase 1: Crisis
- **Medical** – Onset of disease triggers a crisis → seek relief through medical diagnosis and treatment.
- **Patient** – Shock, disbelief, disorientation, mood swings, isolation; external locus of control and external locus of treatment.
- **Family** – Family and caregivers experience disbelief, revulsion, and rejection.
- **Basic task** – Deal with symptoms, pain, or traumas.

Phase 2: Stabilization
- **Medical** – Plateau of symptoms is reached, and individuals become more familiar with their illness.
- **Patient** – Attempts pre-illness activity level → overtaxes and contributes to relapses and the ensuing feeling of upset and failure.
- **Family** – Family expects patient to return to past responsibilities → disappointment and anger because patient does not resume prior responsibilities and success → divorce or stop support and assistance.
- **Basic task** – Accept illness and comply with treatment regimen; stabilize and restructure life patterns.

Phase 3: Resolution
- **Medical** – Plateaus of symptoms and relapses, but patient better understands illness pattern and others' reactions.
- **Patient** – Existential question: why should patient live and how?; internal locus of control and internal locus of treatment; begin to accept that one's pre-illness self will not return.
- **Family** – Family begins to accept patient pre-illness self will not return and adjusts expectations of the patient; patient reconsiders or develops new friendships and significant others.
- **Basic task** – Patient and family grieve loss of pre-illness → self-awareness and options to develop a new self and meaningful philosophy of life and spirituality.

Phase 4: Integration
- **Medical** – Some patients experience continuous plateau or even improvement while others worsen.
- **Patient** – Integrates parts of pre-illness self into new self despite plateaus/relapses.
- **Family** – Family, friends, and significant other if possible; reduced or alternative work is sought; if on disability may seek to volunteer; but insist that what they do will be meaningful.

- **Basic task** – Find appropriate employment; if on disability find volunteer activity; or live meaning fully; reintegrate or form supportive networks of friends and family; further integrate one's illness within a spiritual or philosophical framework.

There are many strengths to adopting this model as a framework for treating chronic illness. One of the primary ones is that it accounts for the complex nature of chronic illness. Individuals may not progress in a stepwise and sequential manner. Life, individuals, and their illness course present as a very complex and interrelated set of systems. The complexity of the individual, the course of their illness, and the context of their life present many variables to the clinician. This model allows for such ambiguity and complexity as clinicians guide the individual toward increases in functioning and quality of life.

A second strength of this model is that it provides a framework of understanding for individuals who cycle between the stages at different times. This movement can be viewed as maturity and practice, as opposed to regression to an earlier/previous stage. This allows the clinician to consistently adopt a flexible and strength-based approach.

A third strength of the model is the outlining of tasks for the individual to address in order to improve their functioning and quality of life. The tasks are appropriate to the individual's development in coping with their illness. This provides a clear framework of understanding and can guide the clinician in targeted interventions.

A fourth strength is that the model incorporates and addresses the individual's community and support system, including family, friends, and work environment. Many individuals struggle with inadequate or ineffective support systems. The model addresses common reactions among such systems, from assessment to setting the stage for psychoeducation or direct therapeutic intervention.

Notes to clinicians and individuals

- It is important to be familiar with the stages of cancer, since they provide context and information about the individual seeking services. Each stage has unique challenges, and needs, wants, and concerns vary greatly among them.
- It is important to have a conceptual framework for understanding chronic illness and the complexities that individuals present with. Fennell's (2003) four-phase model does a great job of outlining the challenges, needs, and potential points of clinical intervention and integrates well with all psychological theories and skills-training approaches.
- I strongly encourage the treating clinician to become familiar with the four-phase model and to read its source material in order to gain a better understanding of its basic assumptions and complexities.

Biological Curriculum

Session focus: Increased functioning and quality of life

TAG
Teach – Apply – Generalize

- The goal of this session is to:
  - Create a baseline of functioning
  - Establish the individual's view of their quality of life
- What to discuss:
  - Defining functioning and the need for assessment
    - Addressing barriers to functioning
  - Defining quality of life
    - Addressing barriers to quality of life
  - The importance of making efforts to improve one's life
- Skills to teach:
  - Assessment of the individual using the SCL-90-R or other tools
  - Assessment of the individual using the Quality of Life Questionnaire or other tools
- Generalize:
  - Create an action plan to assess and discuss the individual's functioning and quality of life
  - Problem-solve barriers
  - Commit to the individual's plan and review results
- Review goal sheet

Increased functioning and quality of life

Introduction of the topic

Functioning

This session is designed to orient the clinician to assessing for functioning. Individuals who experience a chronic and potentially life-changing illness struggle with functioning in many areas of their lives. Assessment can provide the individual and the clinician valuable information to guide clinical interventions, participate in treatment planning, and create a baseline of functioning to track progress over time. The focus of assessment is on the individual's needs. This involves gathering information on their functioning in relation to survival and maintenance of their current functioning in the light of the multitude of challenges that a chronic illness may present. Some of the areas to assess include:

- How has the individual learned to live with the physical effects of the illness?
- How do they cope with the treatments of the illness itself?

- Does the individual communicate effectively with doctors?
- Are they able to maintain emotional stability when coping with intense feelings?
- Are they able to challenge the demoralization process?
- Do they understand the condition?
- Do they need further education about the treatment and therapy?
- Do they have the skills to build trust and confidence in the doctors, especially when recovery isn't possible?
- Are they effectively engaging in symptom management?
- How do they manage social relationships when faced with an uncertain medical future or when symptoms arise?
- Do they struggle with social isolation?
- How effectively do they manage chronic stress?

Think of assessment as a process. You are initially gathering information in order to assess the individual's needs and functioning. Strengths and areas of vulnerability will emerge. Assessment tools and interview questions can help establish the initial areas of functioning to address clinically. As the individual progresses in therapy, the assessment tools can provide ongoing information about progression, stagnation, or regression. All of these possibilities are potential targets for clinical intervention. Some clinicians fail to share the assessment information with the individual. This is a potentially grave mistake. The individual will feel disenfranchised and will not be a leader in their treatment team. This is counter to what we want when engaging in evidence-based practice. Share the results in real time as points of discussion and provide information that can guide the therapeutic process. This is standard of practice in EBPP.

It is important to identify which tools to use and when to use them. A suggested practice is to use a combination of tools throughout the course of therapy. Here are a few examples of how assessment tools can be used:

- **Example 1** – It is common to use one tool in the initial assessment and the same tool at the end of therapy. This establishes a pre–post measurement on therapeutic outcomes. This is typically done when the assessment measure is rather large (items) and time-consuming (length). You may need to consider the financial impact of the length of administration, the cost of the tool, licensing agreements, the ability to bill for the services, and ease of use.
- **Example 2** – Identify one tool to use throughout the entire course of treatment, administered at meaningful intervals. Using one tool throughout the process can assist in establishing pre–post measurement, while providing consistent information across administrations. The strengths of using one tool are consistency (for both the clinician and the individual) and the ability to aggregate data. Potential drawbacks include a "practice effect" for the individual when reporting through the tool, either too global or too specific outcomes, and loss of therapeutic value over time.
- **Example 3 (recommended)** – Take a hybrid approach in combining the previous options. Identify one tool for a pre–post measurement that tends to be quite global in assessing an individual's functioning across multiple domains. Use a separate

tool to track a more limited number of domains in order to gather more specific and sensitive information, with specific time intervals between administrations. You can change tracking tools throughout the therapeutic process in order to assess different areas of functioning that are more sensitive to the changing needs and abilities of the individual. Track the individual's functioning through one tool until a separate tool is needed to assess a different set of domains. This provides a high degree of flexibility in the assessment and outcome tracking process. There are a few things to be cautious of when adopting this approach. Be careful to establish intervals that are not too close together, or you will continually assess the same information without allowing time to change. It can be problematic to use too many tools, as the information being gathered may lose meaning. Identify a few tools that are easy to use, provide meaningful data, and assess the domains you want to target.

There are many strengths to taking this approach in therapy. Having discussions about the need for further information and tracking of progress can be invaluable. Talk openly about the value of information and how it can guide decisions and interventions in therapy. This open dialogue informs the individual about what to expect from the therapist and how to measure success. The approach relies on the strengths of the individual in addressing their areas of growth. Information gathered through the assessment tools provides real-time data to guide the clinician and the consumer. The information can be used to establish both initial and ongoing treatment targets. It is also important to openly discuss the results of the assessment, while balancing sensitive and at times painful information identified through the process. All of the information made available is a point for discussion. Informed individuals tend to be more motivated, more resilient, less hesitant and impulsive, and to have more ownership and compliance throughout the process.

Quality of life

The Centers for Disease Control and Prevention (2003) defines quality of life as:

> a broad multidimensional concept that usually includes subjective evaluations of both positive and negative aspects of life. What makes it challenging to measure is that, although the term "quality of life" has meaning for nearly everyone and every academic discipline, individuals and groups can define it differently. Although health is one of the important domains of overall quality of life, there are other domains as well – for instance, jobs, housing, schools, the neighborhood. Aspects of culture, values, and spirituality are also key aspects of overall quality of life that add to the complexity of its measurement. Health is more than just a means of living longer. The real purpose of health is to allow a more satisfying and meaningful life, to enjoy a higher quality of life…People are living longer with chronic illnesses such as cancer and diabetes. They need help coping with the ways their lives are altered by the disease…Nearly half of the people who get cancer live, and there are many more long-term survivors than in the past…For these people, there are lots of quality of life issues because the cancer itself is difficult, and the treatment is difficult…Whether caused by cancer or chemotherapy, side effects such as pain, fatigue, depression, anemia, impotence, loss of appetite and inability to taste or smell can be devastating.

It is clear that self-perceptions predict mortality, morbidity, and future use of health care services. These are important reasons to assess for quality of life and to work in therapy toward remoralization and building resiliency. Assessment of quality of life has a clear relationship with motivation, compliance, and satisfaction, while having the predictive validity previously mentioned. It is suggested that quality of life be evaluated concurrently with assessments targeting functioning. This allows the clinician to discuss the relationship(s) between functioning and quality of life. It is strongly encouraged to additionally measure satisfaction with services. This can provide very meaningful data on the therapeutic relationship, as well as on the process itself.

Notes to clinicians and individuals

- One of the most important factors to consider when selecting any form of outcome or tracking tool is whether the tool matches the needs of the population being served.
- Incorporate the information gained through the assessment tools in the treatment planning process.
- Be consistent in the administration of measures.
- Inform the individual about your practice regarding assessment measures when you are covering informed consent.
- Research potential billing or contracting mechanisms so you can be reimbursed for your use of the selected tools.
- Informed individuals tend to be more motivated and compliant throughout the therapeutic process.
- Report the results in a manner that the individual can understand, balancing sensitivity with accurate reporting.

Session focus: Goal setting and motivation

TAG
Teach – Apply – Generalize

- The goal of this session is to:
  - Create one goal in each of the three areas: biological, psychological, and social
  - Provide feedback from assessment tools/measures and incorporate this into the feedback and treatment planning process
  - Personalize the client tracking tool for in-session use
  - Learn coping skills to improve the individual's functioning in the areas of goal setting and motivation, in order to allow them to cope in a more effective manner
- What to discuss:
  - Setting realistic goals
  - Balancing wants with needs
  - Maintaining commitment to change
  - Introduction of relevant forms
- Skills to teach:
  - Observe, Describe, Participate
  - Non-judgmental Stance, One-Mindfully, Effectively
  - Radical Acceptance, Practical Acceptance, Practical Change, Radical Change
- Generalize:
  - Create an action plan to complete **Goal Setting** (see handout)
  - Problem-solve barriers
  - Commit to the individual's plan
  - Review in next session
- Review goal sheet

Goal setting and motivation

Introduction of the topic

Many individuals want to make changes in their lives. Change is a natural state that allows individuals to adapt, cope, and find enjoyment in life. Individuals are seldom taught how to be advocates for their own change. They may see something that they want and try to get it. When barriers and difficulties arise, they often try to continue on their current path until they get what they want, or quit trying because they lose hope. There are fundamental aspects to goal setting that are not formally taught. Education programs do not typically teach steps to goal setting. Life experiences tend to be the primary teacher. Individuals learn in a few basic ways, and they can become quite rigid when they are forced to change. It may be easier to do nothing and just accept what is happening. Individuals may feel that what is happening is unjust and respond by fighting against everything. All individuals feel like giving up or fighting everything at times, but extreme reactions tend to be very ineffective. They need to find balance,

Biological Curriculum

flexibility, and perseverance if they are to be effective in a consistent manner. Most individuals struggle in three main areas: setting realistic goals, balancing wants with needs, and maintaining their commitment to change.

Setting realistic goals

There are a few key points to review concerning the process of goal setting. Goals need to be based in reality, and they need to be attainable. Many individuals want a cure from their illness. This is not realistic for most people. Hoping for a cure can often create barriers to coping and eventually decrease the individual's ability and desire to cope with their current situation. They need to strike a balance between hope for improvement (not a cure) and the work needed to increase functioning and quality of life. Chronic health issues can often lead to decreased hope (demoralization) and feelings of disempowerment and inability to necessitate change. Consistent work with goals and objectives can provide the core tools to improve hope and lead to more effective functioning and improved quality of life. There are three main steps to setting realistic goals: identifying the VOR, setting the goal, and establishing stepwise and sequential steps to reaching the goal (objectives).

Balancing wants with needs

Many individuals struggle with prioritizing their work in treatment. It is natural in the course of treatment to want to focus on the most recent crisis, change in health, or change in functioning. This may be very appropriate for many individuals, but can lead to loss of focus for treatment priorities. The clinician and the individual must agree upon the needs of the individual and prioritize treatment targets as a first step. Once that is done, a skills implementation plan can be completed to target crises that may arise without losing focus on the treatment priorities. This allows for crisis work in addition to maintaining focus on the agreed-upon treatment targets as changes occur.

A need in treatment can be defined as something that is necessary to the individual's living a healthy and meaningful life. Needs are distinguished from wants because a deficiency in a need would cause a clear negative outcome, such as decreased functioning or increased vulnerability to painful emotional experiences. A want is simply something that a person would like to have. Most individuals struggle with the wish or desire to return to a life free from physical illness and mental health issues. This is not realistic for most people. Many individuals focus on what they have lost and what they can no longer do. This focus on the past can lead to a variety of painful emotional experiences, resulting in demoralization and loss of hope, and ultimately in compromised focus and follow-through with treatment recommendations. It is a priority to set goals that are based on needs as opposed to wants during the initial stages of therapy. This encourages the individual to focus more on the present and on opportunities for change in the future. A potential therapeutic benefit is an increase in perceived power and control. The process does not necessarily devalue or invalidate the past, but encourages focus on what can be done now to allow the individual to be an advocate for positive change in their own lives.

Maintaining commitment to change

Maintaining commitment to change is very difficult for most individuals experiencing a chronic illness such as cancer. Goals and objectives need to have meaning in the individual's life. The clinician is encouraged to establish treatment targets that are relevant to the individual and that are co-created. If goals and objectives are not relevant or are forced upon the individual, motivation, commitment, and compliance can be compromised. Choosing targets for treatment with the support and guidance of the clinician reinforces a healthy connection without reinforcing tacit agreement by the individual. It may also discourage passive compliance, which is a primary barrier for many individuals. It is important to remember that many individuals have had very little choice in their treatment and procedures, or in the effects that cancer and mental health issues have had in their lives. Consult with the individual to agree on initial targets for treatment and for progression in therapy throughout the review process, while continuing to track outcomes in functioning and quality of life.

Flexibility is another key concept to review with individuals. It is important to challenge all-or-nothing thinking and looking at the world through a black-and-white lens. It is valuable to understand that much of life is lived and experienced between "the opposing poles of certainty." When individuals are forced to change, it is natural for them to want to simplify a very complex process and view life through extremes. A problem arises when extreme views no longer serve a primary protective function and become a barrier to change. Extreme views do not lend themselves well to modification and generalize very poorly to most aspects of life. The process traps many individuals into thinking that they need to protect themselves from further unanticipated change, and they become stuck. They are then more vulnerable to rejection, loss of hope, and invalidation. The clinician needs to validate the extremes and that they serve a purpose at times. The individual can be encouraged to accept what is a stepping stone toward advocacy for change. The focus can then be turned to other potential options and the pros and cons of making or not making choices. The goal of flexibility is to provide options and choices that are not accessible to the individual when they are stuck in polarizing extremes.

The last concept for review in this section is the importance of recognizing positives in life. Review the phrase: "keep your nose to the grindstone." This means applying oneself conscientiously to one's work. Many individuals also value having a strong work ethic. They need to be cautious about focusing too much on change and moving away from their emotional and physical pain too quickly. It is important to remind individuals that the change process is like a marathon and not a sprint. There is value in recognizing the existing positives, as well as the positives we are all trying to create in our lives. If they hyper-focus on distress and change, they run the risk of losing focus and momentum in treatment. It is important to recognize small steps toward a healthier life. Individuals can challenge their perspective by refocusing on what they want to add to their lives instead of what has been lost. Use terms such as "increase" and "gain" instead of "decrease" and "lose." These changes can represent a fundamental shift in thought, behavior, and experience by grounding the individual in the present time.

Teaching skills (T)

The first set of suggested skills to teach is an overview of the mindfulness skills from Linehan's (1997) DBT manual. These skills can assist in pattern recognition, awareness, and identification of coping strategies in need of improvement. These are important concepts in the creation of therapeutic treatment targets and ongoing skills use targeted at increasing effective coping.

- **Observe** – Noticing one's experience.
- **Describe** – The process of putting words on one's experience.
- **Participate** – What the individual is doing to cope with the current situation and how present they are in the process.

When these skills are used in combination or in a liner fashion, they provide a process through which to recognize patterns of thoughts, behaviors, and emotions. They can be used to identify how an individual interprets, reacts, and attempts to cope with an event. This promotes increased awareness of how they typically respond to events. These are key skills in behavioral and cognitive analysis.

- **Non-judgmental Stance** – Noticing our experience without placing value (right/wrong and good/bad) on the experience itself, or on the process.
- **One-Mindfully** – Focusing our attention on the present situation or task.
- **Effectively** – Doing what is required to meet needs in a healthy manner.

When these skills are used in combination with the previous ones, it can provide awareness regarding the effectiveness of the individual's attempts to cope, and can essentially provide a baseline of functioning from which to start the treatment-planning process.

Acceptance versus change

Linehan (1997) introduced the concept of dialectics, involving a balance of acceptance and change to assist individuals in coping more effectively with difficulties in their lives. Acceptance is the process of acknowledging something without attempting to change it. It is not about quitting or giving up, but rather recognizing the reality of a situation. The reality of the individual is often an effective starting point for engagement in the therapeutic process. Many individuals do not want to accept their current situation and want everything to change. This can lead to unrealistic goals and expectations. Conversely, if they accept everything, they will do nothing about their current situation and will often end up suffering. A new set of skills will be introduced to target this key concept in treatment, including **Practical Acceptance** (PA), **Practical Change** (PC), and **Radical Change** (RC). These skills are designed to assist in the process of setting realistic goals and guiding the individual through balancing acceptance and promoting healthy change.

    The second set of skills to teach targets the balance between acceptance and change. The concept of dialectics may be defined as a commitment to the core conditions of acceptance and change. Progress is made by combining elements that are opposite to one another in order to create a synthesis based in reality. An example is that I may want to be free from distress (a desire for change), but right now I experience distress on a daily basis (acceptance or what is). If an individual is able to synthesize the truth of both extremes, they have an increased ability to view their experience in a more realistic manner. The synthesis may involve a combination of focusing on one or more of the skills outlined in this section.

Acceptance   Change

|-------------------------------|---------------------------|---------------------------|

Radical Acceptance   Practical Acceptance   Practical Change   Radical Change

On one end of the dialectic is **Radical Acceptance** (RA). This may be defined as accepting reality for what it is. It is letting go of fighting or resisting one's current situation and accepting that attempts to change reality may be futile. It is about accepting 100% of the situation while focusing to change how one copes and adapts to the situation itself. That is where power and perceived control are found. For example, an individual may need to accept that distress is a part of their everyday life and that their current option is to change how they respond to this reality.

A less extreme version of this skill is **Practical Acceptance** (PA). This may be defined as accepting that seeking control of the situation is futile, but still being able to influence the situation. PA encourages the individual to accept the situation for what it is, while understanding they can still change aspects of it and how they respond to it. PA is less extreme than RA in the sense that the individual still needs to accept reality for what it is, but has not exhausted all attempts to influence (change) internal or external factors that are causing distress. This skill allows for a high degree of acceptance, while encouraging appropriate action designed to promote healthy change. The individual may accept 80% (most aspects that are change-resistant) of the situation while targeting 20% (some aspects that can be influenced) for change. For example, an individual may need to accept that their distress is limiting their functioning and that they can still modify their actions and change how they respond to this reality.

The next skill on the dialectic is **Practical Change** (PC). This may be defined as changing many aspects of a situation and needing to accept some aspects that are change-resistant. PC encourages the individual to focus on action and changing the situation itself, while also changing how they respond to it. The skill allows for the promotion of a high degree of change, while encouraging the acceptance that not all aspects will change. The individual may target change for 80% (most aspects that can be influenced) of the situation while accepting 20% (some aspects that are change-resistant). For example, an individual may need to change their activity levels due to physical distress/pain, while accepting some limitations that cannot currently be changed.

The last skill on the dialectic is **Radical Change** (RC). This may be defined as changing all aspects of a situation because no other alternative is acceptable. This is an extreme skill, designed for application in extreme situations. RC is about the individual changing 100% of the situation, while focusing to change how they cope and adapt to the situation itself. This is where power and perceived control are found. For example, an individual may need to change their entire approach to treatment if noncompliance or partial compliance is not effective.

Applying skills and concepts (A)

- Introduce/discuss a **Diary Card**
- Introduce/discuss a **Skills Implementation Plan**
- Introduce/discuss cognitive analysis
- Introduce/discuss behavioral analysis
- Create safety plans and commitment expectations
- Actively create goals and objectives in session
- Discuss common barriers to this process

Generalizing skills and concepts (G)

- Problem-solve barriers to setting treatment goals and objectives
- Create an action plan for **Goal Setting** (see handout)

Notes to clinicians and individuals

- A primary goal is to increase the probability of meeting needs in a healthy manner. One process to consider is how to effectively balance acceptance and change. Exploring potential combinations of these concepts can provide a realistic set of strategies and skills for the individual to apply to their challenges.
- Always lead with strengths, when possible.
- Treatment needs to be viewed like a marathon and not a sprint.
- Skills tend to be most effective when used in combination.
- Three new skills have been introduced to promote healthy coping.
- Treatment goals and objectives are more effective when created *with* individuals, not *for* them.
- Treatment plans gain more acceptance and ownership, and better promote compliance, when shared and coordinated with the entire treatment team.

Session focus: Orientation to change

TAG
Teach – Apply – Generalize

- The goal of Step 1 of this session is to:
  - Gain insight and information about the impact that perceived control has in coping with change
  - Learn coping skills to improve the individual's functioning in the area of coping with change
- What to discuss in Step 1:
  - The definition of "locus of control"
  - The concepts of control and influence
  - How perceived control influences functioning and how it affects approaches to treatment
- The goal of Step 2 of this session is to:
  - Identify where in the change process individuals are, while assessing for motivation to progress and make changes in their lives
  - Learn coping skills to improve the individual's functioning in the areas of motivation and change
- What to discuss in Step 2:
  - Change
  - Distress and overall functioning
  - **Stages of Change** (see handout)
- Skills to teach:
  - Observe, Describe, Participate
  - Effectively
- Generalize:
  - Create an action plan for **Control versus Influence** (see handout)
  - Create an action plan for reviewing/modifying treatment plans
  - Problem-solve barriers
  - Commit to the individual's plan
  - Review in next session
- Review goal sheet

Step 1: Orientation to change

Introduction of the topic
If an individual feels like they have some control in a situation, they are more apt to act and advocate for themselves. If the same individual believes that they have little to no control, they may become quite passive, or even resistant. Every person has tendencies in how they respond to situations. It is important to note that these tendencies are not "right" or "wrong," but only effective for the individual or not. One way of viewing these tendencies is to explore them through the concept of a locus of control (Rotter, 1954).

Biological Curriculum

Orientations

Internal locus of control

An internal locus of control may be defined as the degree to which an individual believes that they can control their own lives. Individuals who have a high internal locus of control believe that they are free to live their own lives, find or create choices to advocate for themselves, and take responsibility for their actions. Freedom, choice, and responsibility are key aspects to improved health.

How a person reacts to change is important to the treatment of both physical and mental health. Change may be planful. An individual can set realistic goals and steps to reach those goals. They can identify strengths to assist them in the challenges that change presents. They can anticipate barriers to change and react accordingly. An example of this might be applying for employment: There are certain steps to take in order to change job status. An individual typically starts this process by researching what jobs are available and whether they will qualify for the application process. They may gather documents, complete an application, schedule an interview, and complete the hiring process. This reaction to change is self-driven, planful, and proactive.

External locus of control

An external locus of control may be defined as the degree to which an individual believes that their decisions and life are controlled by environmental factors that they cannot influence. Individuals who have a high external locus of control believe that they have little freedom in their lives and tend to feel that they are trapped, that others make decisions for them, and that others are responsible for how things affect them.

There are also instances in which change is forced upon an individual. This may not allow for planning before the change actually happens. Individuals are forced into a position where others are more powerful than they are in their own lives, where they are presented with others' plans for them, and where they must react to a situation instead of shape it in a proactive manner. An example of this might be recovering from an injury-related accident: The individual immediately becomes a "patient" or "client" and has a team of professionals who are responsible for providing treatment or services. The professionals have more knowledge and expertise than the individual. They explain options and suggest plans for interventions and care. The individual is forced to react to the situation.

Control versus influence

It is important to identify how the individual perceives control in their lives and how this perception or belief affects their functioning. "Control" may be defined as "having power over something." A common belief is that if a person views themselves as "being in control", they *should* be able to exert their power and force change. This can be very positive when the change that the person desires *can* be made reality through their efforts. A problem arises when the situation or an individual's response is resistant to being controlled. If they attempt to exert their power and do not get the desired result, they become polarized in their interpretation: "I failed," "I needed to work harder or do more." Polarized interpretations lead to all-or-nothing and black-and-white thinking. This reduces freedom of acceptable experience, restricts choices, and makes it difficult for the individual to take responsibility for their actions. This may become clearer through a common example: Many individuals believe that they can "control" their emotions. If emotions could truly be controlled, however, there would be no use for medication-management or psychotherapy: people would simply exert their power and choose not to be depressed or anxious. The belief that things can be controlled implies that there is a clear and predictable course of action that leads to one acceptable outcome. This belief does not generalize well to the reality that most individuals experience.

"Influence" may be defined as "producing some effect without exerting direct control or power." If an individual focuses their attention on exerting influence, they have more choices and possibilities. Influence challenges all-or-nothing and black-and-white thinking. This concept can be clarified by continuing the previous example: Replace the belief that emotions can be controlled with the belief that emotions can be influenced. This change implies that there is no one clear course of action that leads to one acceptable outcome. The individual does not have to be perfect in their approach to a situation, and can accept that change is a process that is at times dynamic and unpredictable. This shift allows for flexibility in beliefs, interpretations, choices, actions, and acceptable outcomes. There is now a range of what is allowable or acceptable, which can make it easier for the individual to take responsibility for their actions and their involvement in the treatment process.

Step 2: Readiness to change

Introduction of the topic
Change is a natural part of life. When individuals are experiencing challenges in their lives due to physical and emotional health, their lives may feel extremely chaotic. In the midst of the chaos, patterns of functioning emerge. It is important to identify these patterns in order to address specific issues instead of targeting aspects that are vague and difficult to identify. A point of discussion is that we experience change whether we want to or not. How individuals react to change is a key clinical issue to target. We may be in different stages of change with each separate issue or even with certain aspects of coping and functioning. An individual's engagement in the treatment process has a direct impact on appropriateness for care, what protocols may be effective, compliance to treatment, and motivation for change. Before this concept is explored in depth, it is important to provide a context for discussion. This can be done by exploring how distress affects overall functioning.

Distress and overall functioning
If an individual is in a state of high distress, they may respond by being reactive, desperate, and impulsive. This leads to a decrease in functioning and effective coping if the distress is experienced over long periods, as in the case of chronic pain and illness. One of the keys of dealing with this concept is to teach the individual skills and to hold them accountable for practicing them. Through consistent skill work, it is anticipated

that the individual's distress will reduce, functioning will improve, and quality of life will increase.

Stages of change

Researchers have identified **Stages of Change** in relation to individuals experiencing chronic pain (Kerns et al., 1997). There are four stages to review in this session:

1. **Precontemplation (not ready)** – The individual embraces beliefs that the pain problem is medical, that medical professionals will relieve it, and that learning self-management skills is useless.
2. **Contemplation (getting ready)** – The individual recognizes the potential usefulness of self-management, but is reticent to abandon the search for a medical cure.
3. **Action (doing)** – The individual accepts the need for a self-management approach, and is encouraged in efforts to acquire new skills in order to enrich existing ones.
4. **Maintenance (relapse prevention)** – The individual has a well-established belief in the usefulness of self-management, and intends to continue consolidating and expanding their skills.

Teaching skills (T)

The sets of suggested skills to teach in this session are designed to increase the individual's ability to identify their readiness and orientation to change. It is important to integrate the two concepts and apply them to both physical and psychological functioning.

- **Observe** – Noticing one's experience.
- **Describe** – The process of putting words on one's experience.
- **Participate** – What the individual is doing to cope with the current situation and how present they are in the process.

This set of skills will provide a pattern of *interaction* that will assist in identifying the individual's locus of control. When these skills are used in combination or a liner fashion, they provide a process for recognizing patterns of thoughts and behaviors. They can be used to identify how an individual interprets, reacts, and attempts to cope with an event. This promotes increased awareness of how an individual typically responds to events.

This set of skills can be used to identify where in the stages of the change process the individual currently is. It is important to separate physical and mental health. First, each individual should identify their current physical abilities and challenges and review their treatment and care plans. This will provide the context for their current participation in their health care. Then, they should do the same thing with regard to their mental health. After this, they can apply the skill of **Effectively**.

- **Effectively** – Doing what is required to meet needs in a healthy manner.

This skill is important to teach and review when identifying whether the individual's current functioning is optimal or acceptable. Observe, Describe, and Participate provide information about patterns and where the individual is in the change process; Effectively provides information about how effective the individual is being. If what they are doing meets their needs in a safe and healthy manner, the plan should be continued. If what they are doing does not meet these criteria, it should be reviewed and potentially modified.

One way of engaging in this process is to have the individual complete a self-assessment on their current level of functioning in physical and mental health. Then have them review their assessment with their support system and with professionals currently working with them on their care plans. This process is intended to provide points for discussion and challenges to viewpoints, to increase insight, and to coordinate efforts and care. It may also assist the individual in identifying whether their current situation and their responses to it are acceptable and effective for themselves and others, or if modification is needed.

Applying skills and concepts (A)

- Introduce/discuss the handout on **Stages of Change** for both physical and mental health functioning
- Introduce/discuss the homework assignment on **Control versus Influence**
- Have individuals review the model explained in this session and explain it to you or to one another, in order to gain a higher degree of understanding of the terms and concepts
- Problem-solve barriers to this process

Generalizing skills and concepts (G)

- Problem-solve barriers to continuing or modifying the individual's coping and care plans
- Review the level of engagement in the individual's treatment with their support system and with professionals

Notes to clinicians and individuals

- Changing the individual's locus of control is *not* the goal of this session. It is designed to review their functioning and increase their effectiveness in getting their needs met in a safe and healthy manner, through skill application.
- Challenge all-or-nothing and black-and-white thinking by identifying when it provides a barrier to freedom of experience, restricts choices, and makes it difficult to take responsibility. Explore healthy alternatives.
- Validate that there are times when external factors are more influential and powerful than the individual.
- Perception is reality – keep this in mind when working with individuals who feel stuck in behavior patterns and have difficulty identifying options and potential for change.

Biological Curriculum

- It is important for individuals to understand that distress reduces their ability to cope and function effectively.
- Distress and functioning have an inverse relationship.
- Different individuals in a group may be at different stages of change with regard to each issue, or aspects of issues.
- This work leads to increased insight, motivation, and hope.

Session focus: Working with your team

TAG
Teach – Apply – Generalize

- The goal of this session is to:
  - Increase self-advocacy in an effective manner
  - Gain information and insight into working with multidisciplinary teams
  - Learn coping skills to improve the individual's functioning in the area of working with professionals
- What to discuss:
  - Working with your team
  - Preparing for appointments
  - Engaging in complaining behaviors
- Skills to teach:
  - **Preparing for an Appointment** (see handout)
  - **KEEP IT REAL** (see handout)
- Generalize:
  - Create an action plan for **KEEP IT REAL**
  - Problem-solve barriers
  - Commit to the individual's plan
  - Review in next session
- Review goal sheet

Working with your team

Introduction of the topic
It can be very important for an individual to know the primary functions of a medical appointment from a medical provider's perspective. This can assist them in preparing for an appointment and anticipating the goals and practice of the provider.

According to Goold & Lipkin (1999), there are three main functions of a medical appointment:

- Determine and monitor the nature of the problem
- Develop, maintain, and conclude the therapeutic relationship
- Carry out patient education and implementation of treatment plans

It can also be beneficial for the individual to know that it is challenging for medical professionals to deliver "bad news." There are suggested steps for medical providers to follow, but it may not be common practice for them to adopt a specific protocol when presenting challenging information. In 2000, an article was presented in the *Oncologist* outlining a suggested protocol for medical providers to assist them in this process (Baile et al., 2000). This protocol is named "SPIKES" and consists of six steps:

1. **Setting up the interview** – Mental rehearsal is a useful way of preparing for stressful tasks. This can be accomplished by reviewing the plan for telling the

individual and for how to respond to the individual's emotional reactions or difficult questions.

2. Assessing the individual's **P**erception – Steps 2 and 3 are points at which to implement the axiom "before you tell, ask." That is, before discussing the medical findings, use open-ended questions to create a reasonably accurate picture of how the individual perceives the medical situation – what it is and whether or not it is serious.

3. Obtaining the individual's **I**nvitation – While a majority of individuals express a desire for full information about their diagnosis, prognosis, and the details of their illness, some do not.

4. Giving **K**nowledge and information to the individual – Warning the individual that bad news is coming may lessen the shock that can follow the disclosure of bad news and may facilitate information processing.

5. Addressing the individual's **E**motions with empathic responses – Responding to the individual's emotions is one of the most difficult challenges of breaking bad news. Individuals' emotional reactions may vary from silence to disbelief, crying, denial, or anger.

6. **S**trategy and **S**ummary – Individuals who have a clear plan for the future are less likely to feel anxious and uncertain. Before discussing a treatment plan, it is important to ask the individual if they are ready for such a discussion. Presenting treatment options to individuals (when they are available) is not only a legal mandate in some cases, but will establish the perception that the physician regards the individual's wishes as important.

This information highlights the importance of working effectively with professionals who are part of the individual's care. Understanding how their doctor is preparing to address issues or concerns will allow them to be better prepared for any appointment. There are two topic areas to discuss with individuals to assist them in this process: preparation for appointments and engaging in complaining behaviors. These areas can be barriers to receiving effective care, but can be navigated effectively when done in a thoughtful and planful manner.

Preparation for appointments
Individuals experience many barriers when preparing for medical appointments. There may be delays in scheduling from the time that a need arises to the actual time of the appointment. This delay can lead to an individual forgetting to attend the appointment or forgetting why the appointment was scheduled in the first place, and to changes in symptoms and needs over time. The day of the appointment may also be chaotic due to transportation, childcare, and the weather. Individuals struggle with presenting clear and concise information to professionals. Global and generic languages are often used to describe what an individual is experiencing. This leads the professional to make inferences and assumptions that may or may not be accurate. Another area that individuals struggle with is identifying clear goals and objectives for each appointment. When the structure and process of the appointment are left to the responsibility of the professional, the individual may not get their needs and wants met.

Engaging in complaining behaviors

It can be demoralizing to be in different forms of pain, discomfort, and fear on a daily or weekly basis. It is natural to become frustrated with the process itself and with providers. Many appointments start with the individual discussing their struggles and frustrations. It is important to understand our natural reactions when dealing with someone who is frustrated: it is normal to become defensive, mirror their emotional state, and have a strong desire to distance ourselves from the perceived negativity. Compare this situation to someone working in the lost-luggage department at an airport terminal. People who have lost their luggage tend to use negative language, make demands, or have requests that cannot immediately be fixed, and this puts pressure on the worker to act quickly in a situation that takes time to understand and resolve. There is a lot of pressure to perform, which leads to high burnout rates and high job turnover. It is important for individuals to remember that professionals have a job to do and that they can influence how others treat them. Once an individual has been identified as a "complainer," it is a hard label to change.

Teaching skills (T)

The set of suggested skills to teach in this session is designed to increase the individual's ability to work with professional team members in an effective manner.

Preparing for appointments is a very important activity. The individual can structure a set of tasks to complete before the day of the appointment.

1. **Prioritize needs and wants** – Brainstorm a sheet of needs and wants. Organize them into a list, with priorities at the top.
2. **Set clear goals and objectives for the appointment** – Know the purpose of the meeting and, specifically, what you want to accomplish before the meeting ends.
3. **Create a list of questions for the professional** – Organize your thoughts into a list of questions. Post them in an area that you frequently spend time in so you can add questions to the list as you think of them.
4. **Organize the tracking forms and tracking cards** – Gather the most recent and relevant information you have. This is one way to avoid being forgetful or vague.
5. **Plan for childcare, if needed** – Ask a friend, family member, or the professional's facility to assist. It is important to be able to focus your attention and be mindful during the appointment.
6. **Plan or coordinate transportation** – Make sure you have a reliable plan and mode of transportation. This is one of the main reasons individuals miss appointments.
7. **Plan for an advocate to attend, if needed** – You may want to ask a friend or family member to take notes during the appointment.
8. **Visualize the appointment** – Imagine yourself staying focused, active, and productive in the meeting. This will help increase your chances of meeting your needs.

Structuring the day of the appointment can assist in this process as well.

1. **Confirm childcare** – Avoid last-minute chaos when possible.
2. **Gather materials** – Do not leave them at home.

3. **Review the goals and objectives for the appointment** – Remind yourself of the reasons for the appointment and what you want to accomplish.
4. **Engage in a stress-management exercise** – Take some time to relax and breathe before the appointment. Deep breathing, progressive muscle relaxation, and imagery can help to calm your nerves.
5. **Leave at an appropriate time** – Plan to be about 10–15 minutes early to your appointment. Being late can compromise your chances of having a productive appointment.

During the appointment, remember to **KEEP IT REAL**.

1. **K**eying in on the task at hand – You are attending an appointment with a professional. Be respectful and take an active role in your care.
2. **E**stablish the goals for the appointment – State your goals at the start of the appointment. This will make it clear that you are taking an active role in your treatment and may help in structuring the appointment.
3. **E**stablish the available time – Ask the professional how long they *realistically* will be in the appointment with you and pace yourself accordingly.
4. **P**rovide information – Present your tracking tools and the information you have gathered. This may also include your written list of questions. Be clear and specific.
5. **I** statements – Make consistent "I" statements and take responsibility for your decisions and care.
6. **T**ake notes – Write down the answers to your questions in order to help remember them. You can also review them later.
7. **R**equest written materials – Gather as much information as you can. Information helps with making decisions and motivation.
8. **E**ngage in reflective communication – When a question is answered or you need clarity, let the professional know what you heard and check to make sure your interpretation and memory are accurate.
9. **A**sk questions – Be assertive. No question is too silly or stupid to ask. Do not leave the appointment with unanswered questions.
10. **L**eave with a clear care plan – Know the next steps in your care and discuss them with the professional before leaving.

The next set of skills, from Pederson & Pederson (2012), is designed to help individuals avoid overcomplaining to professionals. It include **Grounding Yourself** (GY), **Willingness** (W), and **Non-judgmental Stance** (NJS). The combination of these skills may help the individual stay focused on their goals, increase their options, and challenge the role of judgment in their current situation.

- **Grounding Yourself** (GY) – Remain in the here and now through the use of grounding exercises. This skill can be used to remind the individual to focus on their goals, be respectful, and be reasonable. Focus the individual's attention on the current situation and what behaviors are required in the moment.

- **Willingness** (W) – Meet others and situations where they are instead of where we wish they were. This skill can be used to challenge all-or-nothing thinking. It encourages the individual to be open to all options that are being discussed.
- **Non-judgmental Stance** (NJS) – Understand when to use judgments and when to let them go. This skill can be used to challenge the individual's view of things as "right" or "wrong" and "good or "bad." Judgments lead to rigid thinking and to acting on emotions that do not to fit the facts of the situation. Look for shades of grey in order to explore potential options.

Applying skills and concepts (A)

- Introduce/discuss the homework assignment on **Preparing for an Appointment**
- Discuss **KEEP IT REAL** (see handout)
- Roleplay attending an appointment
- Problem-solve barriers to this process

Generalizing skills and concepts (G)

- Problem-solve barriers to creating a plan for attending an appointment
- Introduce and assign homework on the individual's appointment plan

Notes to clinicians and individuals

- Remind individuals to help their team help them.
- Being prepared for an appointment increases the probability of meeting wants and needs.
- Remind individuals to be as specific as possible when completing their tracking cards and conveying information to health care professionals.
- Keep a file of treatment protocols and tracking tools that can be shared with the entire treatment team.
- Do not assume that all members of the treatment team have all the information they need to make decisions.
- Treating others respectfully encourages them to treat you in the same manner.
- Be cautious of making emotion-based decisions. Such decisions tend to be impulsive and focused on meeting short-term needs at the risk of damaging long-term relationships.
- Remind individuals to thank their team for participating in their care.

Biological Curriculum

Session focus: Adherence to treatment protocols

TAG
Teach – Apply – Generalize

- The goal of this session is to:
  - Establish the individual's level of adherence to treatment protocols
  - Assess the individual's strengths and barriers to adherence
  - Learn coping skills to improve the individual's functioning in the area of adherence to treatment protocols
- What to discuss:
  - Adherence to treatment protocols
  - Medication adherence
  - Frustration with treatment providers
  - Lack of information
  - Self-advocacy
- Skills to teach:
  - DEAR MAN
  - GIVE
  - FAST
- Generalize:
  - Create an action plan for **Self-Advocacy** (see handout)
  - Problem-solve barriers to adherence to treatment protocols
  - Commit to the individual's plan
  - Review in next session
- Review goal sheet

Adherence to treatment protocols

Introduction of the topic
Adherence to medical treatment protocols may be defined as the extent to which a person's behavior corresponds with agreed recommendations from a health care provider. Research indicates that up to 60% of individuals who are working on a treatment regimen for chronic conditions demonstrate nonadherence to treatment protocols. The implications of nonadherence include lack of progression in treatment, increased costs of health care, loss of productivity and revenue, overutilization of emergency services, increased unnecessary doctor visits, and failure to make lasting changes in functioning.

It is unrealistic to expect every individual to follow the agreed-upon treatment protocols 100% of the time. There are many barriers that lead to nonadherence, which can be broadly separated into four categories for ease of review and discussion.

Medication adherence
According to the Centers for Disease Control and Prevention (2011), adherence is "The patient's conformance with the provider's recommendation with respect to

timing, dosage, and frequency of medication-taking during the prescribed length of time." This definition implies that the patient has a choice and that both patients and providers mutually establish treatment goals and the medical regimen. Medication adherence usually refers to whether patients take their medications as prescribed (e.g., twice daily) and whether they continue to take a prescribed medication. Medication adherence behavior is therefore divided into two main concepts: compliance and persistence. Although conceptually similar, "compliance" refers to the patient's passive following of provider's orders, whereas "persistence" refers to the duration of time for which the patient takes medication, from initiation to discontinuation of therapy.

According to the American College of Preventative Medicine (2015):

- Overall, about 20–50% of patients are nonadherent to medical therapy
- People with chronic conditions only take about half of their prescribed medicines
- Rates of adherence have not changed much in the last 3 decades, despite WHO and IOM improvement goals
- Overall satisfaction of care is not typically a determining factor in medication adherence
- Adherence drops when there are long waiting times at clinics or long time lapses between appointments
- Patients with psychiatric disabilities are less likely to be compliant

The Centers for Disease Control and Prevention also identifies that:

- 20–30% of medication prescriptions are never filled
- Medication is not continued as prescribed in about 50% of cases
- By 2020, the number of Americans affected by at least one chronic condition requiring medication therapy will grow to 157 million
- Rates of medication adherence drop after the first 6 months
- Direct costs are estimated at $100–289 billion annually
- Improved self-management of chronic diseases results in an approximate cost-to-savings ratio of 1 : 10
- Nonadherence causes 30–50% of treatment failures and 125,000 deaths annually

Many individuals are frustrated with the effectiveness of medications. They have questions over whether the correct medications have been prescribed, the right dosages are being administered, and there is potential for over-reliance on their use. Frustration levels are also high with possible side effects, dependency issues, and interactions between medications. Many individuals feel like they have been prescribed medications that have minimal effects and that they need different interventions to promote lasting change. This is especially true when there are multiple side effects and little to no immediate positive effects of the medication. It has been found that individuals typically underuse, overuse, or abuse their medications when nonadherence is an issue. It is important to raise adherence to medication protocols in order to be able to assess for effectiveness and to tell how medication management can assist in stabilizing and potentially improving global functioning. Key interventions include self-empowerment, challenging ineffective behaviors and beliefs, improving communication, and tracking adherence.

Frustration with treatment providers

It is a very common experience to be frustrated with the professionals involved in the provision of care. Many individuals do not feel as if their providers listen well or understand what they are experiencing. It is common to feel rushed in appointments and to question whether the provider is doing all that they can to provide the best care possible. Many individuals do not feel that providers believe them when discussing their experience of distress or pain and their activity levels. One of the most common experiences is to be frustrated about having little influence in the treatment provided. Many individuals have unanswered questions and receive too little information to make effective decisions. Few individuals feel like they have enough power and control in their treatment. If an individual does not feel like they are involved in their own care, motivation for adherence decreases significantly.

Lack of information

The treatment of cancer is often times very complex and difficult for the individual to comprehend. Treatment regimes may include medication adjustments in timing, frequency amounts, and dosage that are difficult to reconcile with the individual's activities of daily living. It is common to have frequent office visits for assessment, labs, invasive procedures, and routine monitoring, as well as unscheduled visits. Many different treatment providers will interact with the individual, and consistent information-passing and coordinated efforts to inform the individual may not always be met. This is very challenging for both professionals and consumers, and often results in confusion and lack of information. Faced with a lack of information, individuals will typically attempt to educate themselves in some manner, which can be very risky. Internet searches may provide information that is unreliable, not relevant, or only partially relevant, that leads to fear-based thoughts and behaviors, and that fosters false beliefs and assumptions. A lack of information can also lead to inactivity, noncompliance, and apathy. It is important to address these barriers before they occur and as they arise, since the process is quite common to all treatment providers and agencies.

Self-advocacy

An aspect of self-advocacy is being assertive in a healthy manner. This means taking an active role in treatment protocols. Individuals are encouraged to co-create care and treatment plans. It is important to ask questions and gather as much data as possible in order to make informed decisions. The individual may also need to assist in the coordination of their own care. Do not be afraid to ask providers if they are sharing information with one another. Make sure that releases for personal health information (PHI) have been reviewed and endorsed. Know what information can and cannot be shared between providers. The individual is typically in charge of deciding what information can be shared, and with whom. Consent to release and share information is required if the team is to function to its highest potential.

A second part of self-advocacy is being aware of your rights. Every agency is required to have and provide a "bill of rights" (BOR) to each individual seeking service. The BOR includes information on the agency's policy and procedures, responsible authorities, data privacy, funding sources, and grievance procedures. In order to be a strong self-advocate, it is important to know your rights. Individuals are often unaware of how their rights may influence their care. It is a common misperception that everybody has equal access to health care. This is not the case! Individuals need to be aware of what health care is available and what procedures and services their insurance covers. Insurance coverage can dictate what services can be accessed.

One of the most difficult and challenging areas of health care is engaging with multiple providers in an effective manner. Health care professionals are very busy and may not have available time to provide and coordinate all aspects of care. It is imperative that individuals learn self-advocacy skills. One aspect of self-advocacy is being aware of the role that each member has in the treatment team. A typical multidisciplinary team might consist of medical doctors, physician-assistants, nurses, nurse practitioners, physical therapists, occupational therapists, psychiatrists, psychologists, and social workers. Each member of the team has an area of competency and a specific set of skills that they use in the provision of care. It is common for many individuals to make a request in a very skillful manner, and for professionals to be unable to grant the request due to their role capacities and capabilities. They may not have the power, authority, or competency to respond appropriately.

Teaching skills (T)

The sets of suggested skills to teach in this session is designed to increase communication skills and effective participation in medical treatment protocols.

Assertiveness training is a key component of working with medical providers. The first set of skills, **DEAR MAN** (DM), provides an overview of the Interpersonal Effectiveness skills from Linehan's (1997) DBT manual (modified in Pederson & Pederson's (2012) DBT manual). It is designed to teach the individual to increase the probability of getting their wants or needs met.

- **D**escribe – Use Observe and Describe to summarize the situation and identify the facts that support the request or the reason for setting a limit or boundary.
- **E**xpress – Share your beliefs or opinions when relevant or required.
- **A**ssert – Ask clearly for what you want or need.
- **R**eward – Let others know how helping you meet your wants or needs will potentially impact their situation.
- **M**indful – Stay focused on your request and avoid leaving the topic.
- **A**ct confident – Use an assertive tone, have confident body language, make eye contact, and stay calm.
- **N**egotiate – Be willing to compromise to meet your wants or needs.

To apply the skill set of DM, the individual needs to first prioritize their needs. Make sure that the person they are communicating with has the capability to meet the request. Be sure to ask the right person at the right time. Consider whether it is appropriate to ask for something given the status of the current relationship. It is also important to review whether the request meets short- or long-term wants/needs.

This is an important skill set to apply in addressing barriers to adherence. It can assist an individual in advocating to be an active member of their own treatment team and viewing themselves as a partner with their physicians and service providers. This promotes working together as a team toward a common goal. It promotes active participation and a sense of empowerment and ownership. The individual could make a request for clear *written* medication instructions that reduce the risk of underuse, overuse, and abuse. These are all key factors in improving adherence.

The skill set of **GIVE** (G) is designed to teach the individual to build and maintain relationships.

- **Gentle** – Be respectful in your approach and avoid threats, demands, and attacks.
- **Interested** – Listen to the other person and be open to the information they have to provide.
- **Validate** – Acknowledge and attempt to understand the other person's perspective.
- **Easy manner** – Be political and treat others in a kind and relaxed manner.

This is an important skill set to apply in addressing barriers to adherence. The effectiveness of one's medical treatment depends partly on the interpersonal context in which it takes place. It is important to have a healthy working relationship with the entire treatment team. A wide body of research suggests that a stressful interaction with the individual's physician tends to have a negative impact on overall health and care. The effectiveness of the individual's care management is influenced by interpersonal styles, the unique interaction the individual has with their physician, and the physician's background, training, and personality.

The skill set of **FAST** (F) is designed to teach the individual how to have self-respect and self-worth.

- **Fair** – Be fair to yourself and others.
- **Apologies** – Do not engage in unneeded apologetic behavior.
- **Stick to values** – Use your own value system as a guide for your behavior.
- **Truthful** – Be honest and accountable to yourself and others.

This is an important skill set to apply in addressing barriers to adherence. An individual who struggles in this area tends to be passive in their treatment, hesitates to discuss any concerns, does not engage in self-advocacy, does not see themselves as a member of their own treatment team, and lacks motivation for positive change and for advocating for their own needs.

Applying skills and concepts (A)

- Discuss DM, G, and F in relation to current adherence levels
- Practice the skills through roleplays
- Problem-solve situations in which one skill might be more effective than the others

- Practice discussing the information gathered through the tracking tools to prepare for future medical appointments
- Practice asking for clarifying information
- Practice taking a more active role in treatment
- Discuss common barriers to these skills

Generalizing skills and concepts (G)

- Problem-solve barriers to medication compliance
- Problem-solve barriers to taking an active role with the current treatment team
- Problem-solve barriers to medical treatment protocols
- Problem-solve barriers to building and maintaining relationships with health care professionals
- Complete and discuss the **Self-Advocacy** homework

Notes to clinicians and individuals

- It may be difficult to prioritize one skill over another. These skills are most effective when applied in combination. The individual may need to start with one skill and then switch to focusing on another in order to meet the demands of the situation.
- Being skillful means increasing the probability of meeting needs – it does not guarantee a positive outcome.
- The simple act of asking questions and fully understanding treatment protocols is an act of self-advocacy. Taking an active role in treatment leads to empowerment.
- Individuals are experts on and about themselves. Fear, anxiety, and depression may lead them to forget this fact.
- The skills taught in this section take time to become effective.
- Practice is required to build proficiency.

Session focus: Pain

TAG
Teach – Apply – Generalize

- The goal of this session is to:
  - Gain insight and understanding into patterns and coping strategies targeting the emergence and ongoing issues/symptoms of an individual's distress
  - Learn coping skills to improve the individual's functioning in the areas of pattern recognition and coping with distress
- What to discuss:
  - Emergence of physical pain
  - Emergence of psychological distress
  - Frequency, intensity, duration
- Skills to teach:
  - **Baseline Assessment** (see handout)
  - Building Mastery, Building Positive Experiences, Mood Momentum
- Generalize:
  - Create an action plan for the **Skills Implementation Plan** (see handout)
  - Problem-solve barriers
  - Commit to the individual's plan
  - Review in next session
- Review goal sheet

Pain

Introduction of the topic
Every individual's pain story is unique, but most share common elements. Our stories typically involve a change in functioning due to a medical condition (cancer diagnosis), an injury, genetics, environmental factors, or a combination of triggers. It is important to reflect on how the individual initially attempted to cope with their pain and what they are currently attempting to do. It may not matter to the individual *how* the pain started, because this cannot be controlled – it tends to matter *that* the pain started and has not ended. Pain affects all aspects of an individual's life. It affects how they think, feel, and act. It affects their attention, concentration, memory, relationships, and physical abilities. Individuals will be strongly motivated to escape their pain, avoid it in some manner, or alter their experience of it. Pain can affect the way an individual thinks, as well as their personality. People can experience automatic negative thoughts, can have a decreased ability to attend, concentrate, and remember, and can become highly pessimistic. Emotional reactions typically include anger, frustration, demoralization, and apathy. Pain can lead to changes in behavior, including inactivity, avoidance, argumentativeness, substance abuse, and desperate actions. All of these potential reactions leave the individual vulnerable and needing more information about their changes and how they can cope in a new and more effective manner.

An individual may be predisposed (genetically) to develop a certain condition or disorder. This may be the case in more progressive diseases or conditions that have pain as a component, such as the different forms of cancer. In other cases, environmental factors may be the source of an individual's pain. This might be the case in an injury or medical complication. In either case, the individual learns how to cope with their condition over time. We learn how to cope through our own attempts, by modeling the behaviors of those around us, through the mass media, and through the instruction of professionals. Seldom have individuals been taught how to cope in a systematic manner.

It is important to note that pain is a natural part of life. It serves to motivate the individual to withdraw from damaging situations, to protect a damaged body part while it heals, and to teach the individual to avoid similar experiences in the future. We are genetically engineered to withdraw from and avoid pain (e.g., we automatically pull our hand away from a hot stove, without thinking about it). We learn from our experiences with pain, typically in an episodic or chaotic manner. Most people are in pain quite infrequently and do not have a lot of opportunities to practice effective coping techniques. We engage in life, and when we experience pain, we focus on it to try to make it go away. When the pain does not disappear, we are forced to attend to it daily and not episodically. This is a crucial shift to understand: because the pain is present on a daily basis and we do not have many coping techniques to deal with it, we try some random strategies and find something that works for a short period of time. We then tend to try that same coping technique as a first resort and begin to rely on its being effective. Seldom, however, does one technique work for all kinds and levels of pain. Therefore, we create a pattern of responses that works at times and fails miserably at others. This leads to a reinforcement schedule that is intermittent and very difficult to change, resulting in more pain, loss of hope, demoralization, and mental health issues. It creates and feeds a vicious cycle that is very difficult to break.

Issues with mental health and chronic pain provide many challenges to an individual's functioning. The impact is typically experienced on a daily basis. It is important to explore the question, "What do you get out of having issues with chronic pain?" There may be rewards and reinforcers present that lead to avoidance patterns. Many individuals may be reinforced for not engaging in healthy behaviors because of pain. This can promote a lack of assertiveness and compliance issues. It is important to discuss the key concepts of reinforcement of pain and the reinforcement/punishment of healthy activities. This session is designed to identify patterns in experienced pain and to increase the individual's ability to cope more effectively.

Reinforcement of pain

Positive reinforcement
Many individuals are reinforced for having pain as a part of their daily lives. They may or may not be aware of this reinforcement. Positive reinforcement may be defined as the adding of a rewarding stimulus in order to increase a certain behavior or response. An example would be when an individual is experiencing pain and their support system tends to their needs, which feels good to them. Another might be when others do something for the individual in pain that they would be able to do for themselves. In this case, the individual is reinforced for not caring for themselves and may become more passive and dependant on those around them. Their support system then

Biological Curriculum

begins to get frustrated and resentful while the individual becomes more passive and dependant.

Negative reinforcement

Many individuals also fall into a trap through avoidance and inactivity. Negative reinforcement may be defined as the removal of an aversive stimulus designed to increase certain behaviors or responses. An example of this might be when an individual does not want to mow the lawn and claims that they are experiencing pain which precludes them from doing so, and others complete the task for them. They are reinforced for being inactive through removal of the task of mowing the lawn, which they did not want to do. This may also promote inactivity, passivity, and dependence.

A negative feedback cycle can develop as pain leads to inactivity and inactivity leads to more pain. Ironically, the new pain an individual experiences can result from inactivity and not necessarily from the original pain source. This is an important point, because many individuals combine all pain into one category: the pain that they have lived with for so long. They may not appreciate that the soreness that comes from increased activity after being sedentary is not their original pain, nor does it come from their primary source of pain. Many individuals with chronic pain are physically inactive – a tragic irony, because inactivity is a more dangerous enemy than pain. Pain teaches many people to rest and reduce their activities. It seems only natural, but excessive rest (not using your muscles) may be damaging to an individual: it can cause not only a loss of muscle strength, but also a loss of flexibility and endurance. The way to combat such deficits is through mild exercise. We have learned from many studies in the field of physiotherapy that when you move less, you begin to lose strength in your muscles. We call this "deconditioning." The more you rest, the more your muscles weaken. As time goes on, any activity becomes difficult and causes additional pain. The result of this cycle tends to be increased inactivity, loss of hope, demoralization, depression, increased fears, and anxiety. One of the key concepts for discussion is how the individual wants things to be different, given a realistic appraisal of their current abilities.

Reinforcement/punishment of healthy activities

Individuals who experience pain face many challenges. It is important to discuss how individuals are reinforced for healthy activities. This is where individuals build mastery in their lives, experience a sense of accomplishment and competency, and increase hope. It can take the form of compliance to treatment, follow-through with consistent activities of daily living, and engagement in activities at a frequency, intensity, and duration that is appropriate to their current abilities.

Some individuals may also be in a system or pattern of functioning where they are actually punished for engaging in healthy activities. Punishment may be defined as the adding of an aversive stimulus to decrease a certain behavior or response. An example of this concept might be where an individual is told to stop engaging in an activity that they are safe to engage in out of fear of increasing pain levels or increasing their risk of injury. There are many other examples of how individuals are punished for engaging in healthy activities. It would be a useful discussion point to have individuals generate examples of reinforcement and punishment paradigms in order to ground the individuals in their own experience, provide opportunities for validation and acceptance, and provide motivation for appropriate change.

Loss associated with mental health and pain

Many individuals experience multiple losses associated with their mental health and chronic pain. Such losses are often experienced on a daily basis. Examples include significant changes in daily functioning and decreased participation in activities of daily living, focusing on the past and associated negative changes, loss of hope, and demoralization. To cope with such changes, many individuals avoid engaging in activities or overcompensate for the loss. Either response tends to be extreme and does not match the realistic demands of daily living. It is important to discuss the fact that changes in mental health can be addressed through skills training and practice (see the Psychological Curriculum).

Changes in physical functioning can be viewed through the lens of the difference between three forms of pain. Pain that lasts a long time is called "chronic" and extends beyond the expected period of healing. Pain that resolves quickly when the noxious stimulus is removed or the underlying damage or pathology has healed is called "acute." Pain that comes on suddenly and lasts for short periods of time, and that is not alleviated by the individual's normal pain management, is called "breakthrough." It is important to note that individuals cope differently with different forms of pain. One of the primary issues to discuss is the danger of focusing too much on past functioning and the need to modify current activities. When an individual is ready to focus on their current reality, they are more prepared to identify the role of hope in their lives, and they may be empowered to accentuate and build positive experiences in order to gain momentum for healthy change.

Teaching skills (T)

The first set of skills to teach is designed to target behaviors and activities. The goal is to move toward higher functioning through pattern recognition, engagement in activities, and modification of activities when needed. This session is designed to establish baselines of behaviors, identify coping strategies, and introduce/review tracking forms that will be used throughout the treatment process.

Behavioral mapping

It is important for the individual to recognize that certain activities lead to either an increase or a decrease in pain. The **Location of Pain** handout will be used to establish the individual's daily routine and the role of pain in their lives. The individual is to track their activities throughout the day, how they attempt to cope, levels of pain pre/post-intervention, and the location or source of their pain. This form is to be completed daily and reviewed in the second section of the program day.

Event scheduling

It is important to plan and prepare for events that may present barriers to effective functioning. The **Skills Implementation Plan** is designed to prepare the individual for anticipated activities. It can be used to identify stressful events and create a concrete skills-based plan to promote effective coping. The individual is to complete the plan early in treatment and modify it as they learn and apply coping skills throughout the course of the program. It is common to have individuals identify attempts to cope with stressful situations through a wide variety of strategies. The variations in coping may be categorized into three main areas: fight, flight, and freeze (see next section).

Modifying activities

Many individuals struggle with modifying activities. A key point of discussion is to review the frequency (F) of the activity, intensity (I) of engagement, and duration (D) of involvement. Introduce the concept of altering aspects of FID through attempts at self-regulation and pacing strategies.

"Fight" is a common coping response that may be defined as continuing to participate in an activity until its completion, regardless of the pain that is experienced or produced. Many individuals tend to cope with events by "powering through," disregarding their pain triggers.

"Flight" is a common coping response that may be defined as disengaging from an activity that begins to trigger a pain response. This can be very healthy at times, but it may also lead to stopping an activity out of fear that a pain response may occur.

"Freeze" is a common coping response that may be defined as avoiding any activity that might lead to a pain response. Many individuals even choose to avoid activities that have no history of causing pain.

It is important to introduce a "behavior chain" to assist the individual in identifying their responses to activities that may or may not affect their pain levels. This allows for review of the antecedents, the response of the individual, and the generation of behavioral alternatives that target increases in adaptive functioning.

Building Mastery, Building Positive Experience, Mood Momentum, and instilling hope

The second set of skills to teach targets replacement strategies for ineffective attempts to cope. The goal is to engage the individual in behaviors that lead to an instillation of hope and guard against demoralization.

- **Building Mastery** (BM) – Engaging in activities that have a high probability of success. This allows you to experience a sense of competency and perceived control.
- **Building Positive Experience** (BPE) – Engaging in activities that improve quality of life through the experience of a heightened sense of positive emotions. The more time you spend engaging in positive activities, the less you spend focusing on negative situations.
- **Mood Momentum** (MM) – Noticing and engaging in positive experiences and selecting skills that allow you to stay engaged in the activity. It is common to disengage from positive activities in anticipation that "all good things must end." This skill is designed to foster motivation for positive and healthy change.

The set of suggested skills to teach in this session is designed to improve the individual's ability to cope with predictability and uncertainty. Pain can create chaos in an individual's life. It can be both predictable and unpredictable in the same moment. Unpredictable triggers for pain can be very dangerous to an individual, by encouraging them to avoid and disengage from activities that may be safe and healthy. It is possible to begin to make the unpredictable more predictable through behavioral analysis. If we apply the concepts of frequency (F), intensity (I), and duration (D), we can increase the probability of predicting our pain responses. This can be accomplished in a few steps designed to create an action plan: see **Baseline Assessment** handout.

Applying skills and concepts (A)

- Introduce/discuss a **Diary Card**
- Introduce/discuss a **Skills Implementation Plan**
- Introduce/discuss the **Location of Pain** handout
- Introduce/discuss the homework assignment on **Baseline Assessment**
- Introduce/discuss the homework assignment on **Behavior Chain Analysis**
- Have each individual generate applications of BM, BPE, and MM in their lives
- Discuss common barriers to this process

Generalizing skills and concepts (G)

- Introduce and assign homework on the tracking tools, to be completed and reviewed in the next session
- Problem-solve barriers to completing the tools introduced in this session

Notes to clinicians and individuals

- Applying these concepts is designed to challenge old behavior patterns and generate new and more effective ones.
- It is anticipated that themes of fear, anxiety, and avoidance will emerge. It is important to validate the individual's concerns while focusing on what can be done in the present moment.
- Behaviors are present because they meet needs. Modification is needed when behaviors are extreme responses to situations that do not generalize effectively.
- It is important to validate and learn from the past while focusing attention on how the individual can cope more effectively in the present moment.
- Contingency management is an important concept to review. The goal is to activate behaviors that have a high probability of success.
- The more an individual is able to focus on the positives in their lives, the less time they have to dwell on negatives.

Session focus: Healthy habits and sleep

TAG
Teach – Apply – Generalize

- The goal of this session is to:
  - Learn coping skills to improve the individual's functioning in the areas of building and maintaining healthy sleep patterns
- What to discuss:
  - Cancer and sleep
  - How sleep patterns affect functioning
  - Habits and routines
- Skills to teach:
  - Building a routine
  - Maintaining a routine
- Generalize:
  - Create an action plan for sleep hygiene
  - Problem-solve barriers to **Building/Maintaining a Healthy Sleep Routine** (see handout)
  - Commit to the individual's plan
  - Review in next session
- Review goal sheet

Healthy habits and sleep

Introduction of the topic
Up to half of cancer patients don't sleep well at some point, according to the National Cancer Institute (2014). Sleep disturbances occur in about 10–15% of the general population and are often associated with situational stress, illness, aging, or drug treatment. Physical illness, pain, hospitalization, drugs and other treatments for cancer, and the psychological impact of a malignant disease may disrupt the sleeping patterns of persons with cancer. Poor sleep adversely affects daytime mood and performance. In the general population, persistent insomnia has been associated with a higher risk of developing clinical anxiety or depression.

According to the Cancer Treatment Centers of America (2014):

> Trouble sleeping, also referred to as "sleep disturbance," includes insomnia, restless legs syndrome (RLS) and fragmented sleep. Insomnia is the most common, with up to 80 percent of cancer patients having difficulty falling and/or staying asleep. Cancer patients are twice as likely to experience insomnia as people without cancer.

Why sleep matters

A good night's sleep not only feels good, it has significant benefits for cancer patients. Dr. Laurence Altshuler says "patients need as much vitality and energy as possible to fight their cancer. Sleep allows the body to relax and recoup." Dr. Altshuler is the head physician of the Sleep Lab at Cancer Treatment Centers of America® (CTCA) in Tulsa.

"Without sleep, the body becomes even more stressed, which can interfere with its ability to fight cancer," Dr. Altshuler says. "In fact, lack of sleep can depress the immune system, as well as hamper recovery from major illness or injury."

Why cancer patients have sleep problems

Emotional distress is usually the main reason cancer patients don't sleep well. Think of the toll that a cancer diagnosis alone can take, and it's no wonder that cancer patients suffer from sleepless nights. Uncertainty and fears about the future, along with confronting the big decisions about your treatment, create stress that can hamper sleep.

Veronica Stevens, Naturopathic Oncology Provider at CTCA in Philadelphia, says emotional distress disrupts sleep for about 70 percent of the cancer patients she treats. Emotional distress includes worry, anxiety, depression, and overall stress caused related to family issues and financial concerns.

It is important to note that this session is designed to create a pattern of functioning. This will take time to establish and can be difficult to maintain. Many individuals struggle with sleep and self-cares. Disruptions in sleep can be caused by a variety of issues, from activity levels to poor sleep hygiene. When an individual has difficulty with sleep, they may experience fluctuations in mood, decreases in energy levels, and decreased participation in self-cares, which creates a very destructive cycle. This cycle tends to have a global impact on functioning and may be difficult for the individual to recognize. Management of sleep disturbances that are secondary to mental, medical, or substance-abuse disorders should focus on hygiene and underlying conditions (which are addressed in later sessions). Common treatments include a combination of psychotherapy and medication management.

Teaching skills (T)

Healthy sleep hygiene has many common elements, but what works for one individual may not work as well for another. One of the keys to success is for the individual to experiment and find what behaviors work best for them. The skills taught in this section are separated into two categories: building a routine and maintaining a routine.

Building a healthy sleep routine
There are several elements to building a healthy sleep routine. The individual is encouraged to practice these elements in a consistent manner for at least 1 month.

1. **Go to bed when you are sleepy** – Do not force your sleep. It may be helpful to set a consistent time to start your bedtime ritual that assists in preparing you for sleep.
2. **If you do not fall asleep after 20 minutes, you need to get out of bed** – Find a distraction that does not involve strenuous activity and is short in duration. When

you become sleepy, go back to bed. This may require a commitment to this process over and over until positive gains are achieved.

3. **Get out of bed at the same time every morning** – You really want to minimize exceptions to this concept. Consistency is a stepping stone to healthy habits. The more we make exceptions, the harder and longer we have to work.

4. **Establish a bedtime ritual that helps you prepare for sleep** – Engage in activities that calm the mind and body. Warm baths, scents, meditation, stretching, and reading are all effective examples. Notice that watching television is not on this list!

5. **Keep your bedroom cool, quiet, and dark** – This promotes the 3 C's of sleep – cool, calm, and centered.

6. **Keep to your schedule** – Creating healthy habits takes time and consistency. Over time, you will typically experience deeper, restorative sleep.

7. **Avoid naps if at all possible** – If you must nap, keep it to 10–15 minutes in length.

Maintaining a healthy sleep routine

1. **Bed is for sleep, so minimize other activities done in your bed** – Your bed is for sleep, not talking on the phone, watching TV, eating, or working on the computer.

2. **Minimize or stop caffeine intake after mid-afternoon** – This will assist in keeping you calm and relaxed.

3. **Avoid any alcohol consumption within 6 hours of bedtime** – Alcohol and deep, restorative sleep do not mix well

4. **Avoid big meals or being too hungry before bedtime** – It is important to have balance with hunger around bedtime. If you need to eat, moderation is key.

5. **Avoid exercising 6 hours before bedtime** – Daily exercise is very important but needs to be done earlier in the day.

6. **Have a plan to cope with worry thoughts** – Engage in deep breathing, visualization, or progressive muscle relaxation when agitated. Keep a notepad next to your bed to write your worry thoughts down and address them in the morning (practice letting go).

7. **List strategies to get back to sleep** – Focus on relaxing your body and calming your mind. Engage in a quiet, nonstimulating activity.

8. **Consult your doctor** – It is important to do this before starting an exercise program and in order to assess whether your sleep problems require primary medical interventions.

Applying skills and concepts (A)

- Introduce/discuss sleep as a category on the individual's diary card or tracking cards
- Introduce/discuss sleep as a target area to be covered on the skills implementation plan
- Create a sleep hygiene plan and commitment expectations
- Discuss common barriers to this process

Generalizing skills and concepts (G)

- Problem-solve barriers to creating a plan for sleep hygiene
- Introduce and assign **Sleep Hygiene** homework

Notes to clinicians and individuals

- It is important to discuss how the diagnosis, disease process, and treatment of cancer can all negatively impact sleep.
- Fear and anxiety about the disease and treatment can be a primary barrier to healthy sleep habits.
- Encourage individuals to keep a "thought journal" next to their bed, where they can write down their worries and concerns in order to address them during waking hours. This can assist in challenging rumination during sleeping hours.
- The process of creating a sleep hygiene plan takes time and effort.
- Gaining an increase in quality of sleep is the primary goal.
- There are many barriers that need to be addressed in order for healthy sleep plans to be effective – encourage patience.
- It is common for individuals to be unaware of their sleep patterns and the negative impact that the lack of restorative sleep has on their functioning – encourage them to discuss this concept with their support system and professional team members.
- Most adults need between 7 and 10 hours of sleep each day.

Biological Curriculum

Psychological Curriculum

Session focus: Anxiety

TAG
Teach – Apply – Generalize

- The goal of this session is to:
  - o Identify signs and symptoms of anxiety
  - o Learn coping skills to improve the individual's functioning and quality of life in relation to anxiety
- What to discuss:
  - o The signs and symptoms of anxiety
  - o How anxiety can be a cycle
- Skills to teach:
  - o Reactive sets of skills to stay safe and tolerate the moment
    - Distract the mind
    - Imagery
    - Soothing through the senses
    - Distract with ACCEPTS and Turning the Mind
    - TIP skills
- Generalize:
  - o Create an action plan for **Experiential Mapping** (see handout)
  - o Problem-solve barriers
  - o Commit to the individual's plan
  - o Review in next session
- Review goal sheet

Anxiety

Introduction of the topic

According to the National Cancer Institute (2014), anxiety is often manifested at various times during cancer screening, diagnosis, treatment, and recurrence. It can sometimes affect a person's behavior regarding their health, contributing to a delay in or neglect of measures that might prevent cancer. For example, when women with high levels of anxiety learn that they have a genetically higher risk of breast cancer than they had previously believed, they might perform breast self-examination less frequently. For patients undergoing cancer treatment, anxiety can also heighten the expectancy of pain, other symptoms of distress, and sleep disturbances, and can be a major factor in anticipatory nausea and vomiting. Anxiety, regardless of its degree, can substantially interfere with the quality of life of patients with cancer and of their families, and it should always be evaluated and treated.

Studies indicate that up to 50% of individuals diagnosed with cancer will also meet the *Diagnostic and Statistical Manual of Mental Disorders*, 5th edition (*DSM-V*) diagnostic criteria for anxiety (American Psychiatric Association, 2013). Ranges vary greatly based on age, gender, cancer type, and prognosis. "Anxiety disorder" categorizes a large number of disorders in which the primary feature is abnormal or inappropriate anxiety. Symptoms of anxiety become a problem when they occur without any recognizable trigger or when the situation does not warrant such a reaction. In other words, inappropriate anxiety is when a person's heart races, breathing increases, and muscles tense without any reason for them to do so. It is important to understand that anxiety can present with many different levels of intensity, ranging from a minor inconvenience to incapacitation. Common signs of anxiety include:

- Muscle tension, aches, or soreness
- Feeling on edge or feeling restlessness
- Fatigue
- Irritability
- Difficulty concentrating
- Poor sleep

Anxiety may potentially escalate into a panic attack, as indicated by four or more of the following symptoms (*DSM-V*):

1. Palpitations, pounding heart, or accelerated heart rate
2. Sweating
3. Trembling or shaking
4. Sensations of shortness of breath or smothering
5. Feeling of choking
6. Chest pain or discomfort
7. Nausea or abdominal distress
8. Feeling dizzy, unsteady, lightheaded, or faint
9. Chills or heat sensations
10. Numbness or tingling sensations
11. Derealization or depersonalization
12. Fear of losing control or going crazy
13. Fear of dying

Anxiety as a cycle
A diagnosis of cancer is a life-changing event. It can affect all aspects of who someone is, what they do, how they think, and what they feel. Although reactions vary based on the individual and the diagnosis itself, it may be helpful to provide a model to map the individual's experience in relation to anxiety. The handout on **Experiential Mapping** may assist the individual in understanding their reactions to stressful or anxiety-producing events. *Orientation* refers to the individual's general approach to life (e.g., are they optimistic or pessimistic?). This creates a *predisposition* as to how they experience life stressors (e.g., do they expect life to be happy and filled with joy,

or are they waiting for the next challenging thing that life has in store for them?). Then an *event* occurs, which may challenge their view of the world (e.g., they find a lump upon self-examination). Their world view has a lot to do with how they interpret this information: is it something to be questioned and assessed, or do they already know the answer, and it is dreadful? This can trigger a distinctive physiological response – if the interpretation is one of dread, for example, the response might be panic.

A complex response involves how the individual makes sense of their experience through meaning and pattern recognition. A concerned response can involve needing more information, openly questioning what has been discovered, or being extreme and rigid. This is where a potential confirmation bias needs to be assessed. If the individual is taking limited information to confirm their thoughts/fears, their reaction may no longer be based in fact. This can lead to impulsivity and urges. An effective response might be to have an urge to call their doctor and make an appointment, while an ineffective response might be one of denial or an urge to escape/avoid/alter.

Reactions of emotion vary greatly based on the complex nature of each individual. Concern and fear are typically present for both examples. This leads to behaviors that are designed to actively address their concern, or to escape/avoid/alter their painful emotional experience. The consequences of their action or inaction (both real and anticipated) can be explored. This leads to effects on their orientation. Chronic concerns can lead to major orientation changes. It is important to explore whether this cycle leads to healthy thoughts and behavior patterns or to unhealthy ones. Skill-based interventions can be used throughout this process.

Teaching skills (T)

The sets of suggested skills to teach in this session are designed to increase the individual's functioning by allowing them to effectively cope with anxiety and distress.

The individual has two tasks to complete: stay safe and don't make it worse. These skills are designed to assist in this process. They are designed to reduce high levels of distress and are reactive in nature. They are referred to as "gateway" skills: they can be used to create a path out of high levels of distress where other skills may not be as effective or easily accessible, but they are not designed for problem solving and will only work for a short period of time.

The first set of skills is about distracting the individual from their distress or diverting their attention. This is somewhat similar to avoidance, which is common for many individuals, but has a distinct difference: avoiding is designed to escape a painful experience and not address what caused the distress, whereas distracting involves taking a break from intense emotions until the individual is emotionally stable and can engage in effective problem solving to target the cause of the distress.

- **Distracting the mind** – Engaging in activities that disrupt current thought patterns. This skill can be used to distract yourself from catastrophizing or ruminating. Examples include engaging in rigorous physical activity, working puzzles, and any activity that requires attention and concentration. Create your own list of activities that involve action of the body and mind. Thought stopping is also suggested as a skill to review in this set.

- **Imagery** – Picturing (in your mind's eye) yourself tolerating the distress. This skill can be very effective if you have excessive worry. Imagine yourself being powerful, like a superhero. Tell a story in which you are able to defeat your distress, focusing on how you are able to accomplish the feat and what powers you use. This can provide information to assist you not only in distracting yourself, but also in devising problem-solving strategies.
- **Soothing through senses** – Engaging the five senses to promote a sense of peace and serenity. This skill in very effective in grounding yourself in your current experience, which serves as protection from rumination and fear.
  - **Vision** – Looking at a peaceful scene or painting. Noticing the visual details of what is being seen.
  - **Taste** – Slowly eating a "comfort food" and noticing how each bite touches the lips, how it feels to chew and swallow. Noticing whether the food is sweet or salty, hard or soft…focusing on the details of the experience.
  - **Touch** – Squeezing stress balls, using lotions, hugging soft blankets. Noticing how the sun or wind feels on the skin.
  - **Smell** – Smelling scented candles, potpourri, or anything you identify as pleasurable. Lavender scents tend to be very effective.
  - **Hearing** – Listening to soothing music that mirrors the beating of your heart, such as classical or jazz.

The second sets of skills involves diverting attention: **Distract with ACCEPTS** and **Turning the Mind**.

- **Distract with ACCEPTS** – Accept distress in order to effectively apply distraction skills:
  - **Activities** – Activities assist in decreasing distress and can create positive emotions. Plan activities and do something each day. Doing something is often better than doing nothing.
  - **Contributing** – Do something for someone else. Take a break from your own distress by engaging in others' lives in a positive manner. Smiling, volunteering support or assistance, and listening are all examples of this skill.
  - **Comparisons** – Compare your current situation to a time where you were less skillful and less effective. This can provide perspective to your current situation. You can also compare your situation to someone who has it worse than you do. Validate your experience as you search for healthy perspectives.
  - **Emotions** – Engage in activities or thoughts that create emotions that are different than the painful ones you are currently experiencing.
  - **Push away** – Mentally put the distress in a box on a shelf behind a locked door. Take a break from it now, with the intention of addressing it at a safe point in the future.
  - **Thoughts** – Engage in activities that lead to different thoughts. Read a book or magazine, work a puzzle, or count to 100.
  - **Sensations** – Stimulate sensations that are safe to engage in.

- **Turning the Mind** – Continually refocusing your attention and concentration away from the distress and toward the distraction activity. This may need to be done continually to be effective.

The last set of skills, **TIP**, is designed to create an intense physiological response in order to counteract the experience of extreme distress (Linehan, 2014).

- **T**ip the temperature of your face with cold water – Hold your breath and put your face in a bowl of cold water or put ice packs on your eyes and cheeks (hold for 20–30 seconds and keep the water above 50 °F).
- **I**ntense exercise – Calm your body when it is revved up with emotion by engaging in intense exercise for a short period of time.
- **P**aced breathing – Engage in deep breathing and begin to slow to 5–6 breaths per minute. Breathe out more slowly than you are breathing in.
- **P**aired muscle relaxation – Continue deep-breathing exercises and begin to slowly tense and relax different muscle groups.

Applying skills and concepts (A)

- Introduce/discuss the handout on **Experiential Mapping**
- Review homework from previous session
- Problem-solve barriers to this process

Generalizing skills and concepts (G)

- Problem-solve barriers to creating a plan for **Experiential Mapping**
- Modify the individual's **Skills Implementation Plan** to include the skills mentioned in this session

Notes to clinicians and individuals

- The handout for **Experiential Mapping** can be used for many concerns or targets in therapy. It incorporates thoughts, behaviors, and emotions. Interventions can be applied in each category as well as between categories. Be creative!
- Anxiety tends to be a cycle that traps individuals. Look for the need that anxiety meets as a primary target for interventions.
- Remember that anxiety has a base of fear that has been overgeneralized.
- Skills in this section are survival skills. Remind individuals that their two primary tasks are to stay safe and not make it worse. If they are able to accomplish these tasks, they will see increases in functioning and quality of life.
- The handouts and skills mentioned in this session are key topics for psychoeducation for the individual and their support system.
- Focus on applying the skills taught in session. This will assist the individual in generalizing the skills and using them effectively in times of distress.

Session focus: Depression

TAG
Teach – Apply – Generalize

- The goal of this session is to:
  - Identify signs and symptoms of depression
  - Learn coping skills to improve the individual's functioning in the area of depression
- What to discuss:
  - Rates of depression comorbid with cancer
  - The definition and common signs and symptoms of depressive disorders
- Skills to teach:
  - Safety
  - IMPROVE the Moment
  - Resiliency building
    - Building Positive Experience
    - Building Mastery
    - Just Noticeable Change
- Generalize:
  - Create an action plan for **Scheduling Positive Events** (see handout)
  - Problem-solve barriers
  - Commit to the individual's plan
  - Review in next session
- Review goal sheet

Depression

Introduction of the topic

Symptoms of depression are a common experience for individuals who have been diagnosed with cancer. According to the American Cancer Society (2014), one in four individuals diagnosed with cancer also experiences clinical depression.

According to Heffner (2014):

Research has shown that depression is influenced by both biological and environmental factors. Studies show that first-degree relatives of people with depression have a higher incidence of the illness, whether they are raised with this relative or not, supporting the influence of biological factors. Situational factors can exacerbate a depressive disorder in significant ways. Examples of these factors would include lack of a support system, stress, illness in self or loved one, legal difficulties, financial struggles, and job problems. These factors can be cyclical in that they can worsen the symptoms and act as symptoms themselves.

Common symptoms

Symptoms of depression include:

- depressed mood (such as feelings of sadness or emptiness)
- reduced interest in activities that used to be enjoyed

- sleep disturbances (either not being able to sleep well or sleeping too much)
- loss of energy or a significant reduction in energy level
- difficulty concentrating, holding a conversation, paying attention, or making decisions that used to be made fairly easily
- suicidal thoughts or intentions

Treatment

Treatment can either combine both pharmacotherapy and psychotherapy or utilize one or the other individually. Medications used to treat this disorder include Prozac, Paxil, Wellbutrin, and Zoloft...Psychotherapy is useful in helping the individual understand the factors involved in either creating or exacerbating the depressive symptomotology. Personal factors may include a history of abuse (physical, emotional, and/or sexual), ineffective coping skills, and physical health. Environmental factors involved in this disorder include, among others, a poor social support system and difficulties related to finances or employment.

Prognosis

Major Depressive Disorder has a better prognosis than other mood disorders in that medication and therapy have been very successful in alleviating symptomotology. However, many people diagnosed with this disorder find that it can be episodic, in that periodic stressors can bring back symptoms.

Depressive disorders

Major depressive disorder

According to the *DSM-V*, the criterion symptoms for major depressive disorder must be present nearly every day to be considered present, with the exception of weight change and suicidal ideation. Depressed mood must be present for most of the day, in addition to being present nearly every day. Often insomnia or fatigue is the presenting complaint, and failure to probe for accompanying depressive symptoms will result in underdiagnosis. Sadness may be denied at first, but might be elicited through interview or inferred from facial expression and demeanor. With individuals who focus on a somatic complaint, clinicians should determine whether the distress from that complaint is associated with specific depressive symptoms. Fatigue and sleep disturbance are present in a high proportion of cases; psychomotor disturbances are much less common but are indicative of greater overall severity, as is the presence of delusional or near-delusional guilt.

This disorder is characterized by the presence of the majority of these symptoms:

- Depressed mood most of the day, nearly every day, as indicated by either subjective report (e.g., feels sad, empty or hopeless) or observation made by others (e.g., appears tearful).
- Markedly diminished interest or pleasure in all, or almost all, activities most of the day, nearly every day

- Significant weight loss (when not dieting) or weight gain (e.g., a change of more than 5% of body weight in a month), or a decrease or increase in appetite nearly every day
- Insomnia or hypersomnia nearly every day
- Psychomotor agitation or retardation nearly every day
- Fatigue or loss of energy nearly every day
- Feelings of worthlessness or excessive or inappropriate guilt nearly every day
- Diminished ability to think or concentrate, or indecisiveness, nearly every day
- Recurrent thoughts of death (not just fear of dying), recurrent suicidal ideation without a specific plan, a suicide attempt, or a specific plan for committing suicide

Persistent depressive disorder (dysthymia)

According to the *DSM-V*, the essential feature of persistent depressive disorder is a depressed mood that occurs for most of the day, for more days than not, for at least 2 years. This disorder represents a consolidation of *DSM-IV*-defined chronic major depressive disorder and dysthymic disorder. Major depression may precede persistent depressive disorder, and major depressive episodes may occur during persistent depressive disorder. Individuals whose symptoms meet major depressive disorder criteria for 2 years should be given a diagnosis of persistent depressive disorder as well as major depressive disorder. The diagnostic criteria include:

- Depressed mood for most of the day for more days than not
- The presence, while depressed, of two or more of the following:
  o Poor appetite or overeating
  o Insomnia or hypersomnia
  o Low energy or fatigue
  o Low self-esteem
  o Poor concentration or difficulty making decisions
  o Feelings of hopelessness
- Never being without the symptoms for more than 2 months at a time during the 2 years of the disturbance
- Continuous presence of the criteria for a major depressive disorder for 2 years
- The ruling out of other potential causes
- Significant distress or impairment in social, occupational, or other important areas of functioning caused by the symptoms

Adjustment disorder

According to the *DSM-V*, the essential feature of an adjustment disorder is the presence of emotional or behavioral symptoms in response to an identifiable stressor. Stressors can occur singly or multiply, may be recurrent or continuous, and may affect a single individual, an entire family, or a larger group or community. Some stressors may accompany specific developmental events. Adjustment disorders are associated with an increased risk of suicide attempts and completed suicide. Criteria include:

- The development of emotional or behavioral symptoms in response to an identifiable stressor(s) occurring within 3 months of the onset of the stressor(s). These

symptoms or behaviors are clinically significant, as evidenced by one or both of the following:
  o Marked distress that is out of proportion to the severity or intensity of the stressor, taking into account the external context and the cultural factors that might influence symptom severity and presentation
  o Significant impairment in social, occupational, or other important areas of functioning
- Not meeting the criteria for another mental disorder and not being an exacerbation of a pre-existing mental disorder
- Symptoms not representing normal bereavement
- Symptoms not persisting for more than an additional 6 months beyond the termination of the stressor or its consequences

Teaching skills (T)

The sets of suggested skills to teach in this session are designed to increase the individual's ability to cope more effectively with symptoms of depression. The goal is to have the individual engage in activities that create positive reactions in mood and provide distractions from distress. These interventions are designed to build a life worth living, increase resiliency, and increase moralization. It is important to reorient the individual to their changing reality. It is common for them to view their world as already having been changed. By accepting that their needs and situations are actively changing, they can shift to accepting that life is ever-changing and that they need to cope differently than they have in the past. Accepting reality can then lead to self-validation. This is where individuals can acknowledge the high levels of stress in their lives and that if others were faced with similar circumstances, they would struggle to cope as well. This challenges their perceptions of being alone and "silently suffering."

Safety
The first priority is to assess the individual's safety. If they are experiencing suicidal ideation, this must be addressed before any other issue. If they cannot guarantee their own safety, a psychiatric hospitalization needs to be considered. If they are willing to work on keeping themselves safe, a **Safety Contract** can be initiated. This is also a primary clinical target for the **Skills Implementation Plan**. A clear commitment to safety is a primary requirement for continued therapy.

Coping with high distress
- **IMPROVE the Moment** – Tolerating distress by engaging in "pro-life" activities:
  o Imagery – Imagine yourself not only tolerating your distress, but coping effectively
  o Meaning – Find purpose or a lesson that you can learn from your distress
  o Prayer – Connect to something larger than yourself, to assist you in carrying the burden (connecting with your higher power or something larger than yourself)
  o Relaxation – Engage in an opposite stress response (deep breathing, meditation)

- o **O**ne thing in the moment – Channel attention and concentration toward coping efforts
- o **V**acation – Find a safe way to take a break from the distress (visualization, timeout)
- o **E**ncouragement – Practice new narratives of self-validation and encouragement

This set of skills is designed to increase the individual's ability to tolerate stress in the moment. Skill use connects the individual to their need to cope with changing events, and increases their ability to do so.

Resiliency building
- **Building Positive Experience** (BPE) – Creating or engaging in activities that lead to positive moods. Invite others to engage in activities that are pleasurable (e.g., holding hands, playing with children, going for walks). Find ways to spend enjoyable time with others.

This skill is designed to activate behaviors that serve two distinct purposes. It can lead to positive emotions and nurture relationships, which is the primary goal. This promotes healthy activity and leads to increases in positive moods while including others in positive activities. It can also modify activities that have been avoided or stopped due to the impact of physical abilities or psychological distress. The key is to have the individual modify their engagement in the activity instead of not participating in it at all. Modifying activities can also challenge the individual's patterns of all-or-nothing and black-or-white thinking.

- **Building Mastery** (BM) – Engaging in an activity that promotes a sense of accomplishment or increases the perception of positively influencing your own life.

This skill is designed to activate behaviors that provide the individual a sense of competency and acknowledgment that they can influence their perceptions of their own abilities. This skill can be applied to both solo and group activities. The goal is to engage in activities with a high probability of positive outcomes.

- **Just Noticeable Change** (JNC) – Engaging in a behavior that leads to a change in focus or direction.

This is a "baby-steps" skill, providing a first step toward change. It is designed to change the individual's "threshold" of experience. This helps them identify that small steps can have a big impact on the process of change. The goal is to have them do something different to change their current mood. This does not need to be a positive event – it can be neutral. Many individuals actually practice their current mood (listening to sad music, which makes depressive symptoms worse), whether they are aware of it or not. JNC encourages them to break their thought or behavior cycle by doing something different. Many depressed individuals avoid positive activities because they believe it will not affect their mood, it is too challenging, or they are not worth the positive emotion.

Psychological Curriculum

Applying skills and concepts (A)

- Introduce/discuss the homework assignment on **Scheduling Positive Events**
- Problem-solve barriers to this process

Generalizing skills and concepts (G)

- Problem-solve barriers to creating a plan for **Scheduling Positive Events**
- Have the individual share their plan with their support system for support and commitment

Notes to clinicians and individuals

- JNC is a new skill to introduce that activates different behaviors designed to interrupt negative cycles.
- Orient the individual to life as a changing dynamic grounding them in the moment and away from the idea that life has changed and they are being forced to react. This is a shift toward empowerment.
- Safety is the first priority in treatment.
- Change can be difficult, so engage the individual's support system for assistance early and often.
- It is important to review the skills from the "Anxiety" session, since many of these will work with different forms of emotional distress.
- Identify, validate, and reinforce small changes. They are building blocks for success.
- It is important to review the diagnostic criteria for mental health disorders with individuals. Many will have been diagnosed without being given an explanation as to why.
- Acceptance and self-validation are key starting points for any skills-based intervention.

Session focus: Trauma and retraumatization

TAG
Teach – Apply – Generalize

- The goal of this session is to:
  - Identify signs and symptoms of post-traumatic stress (PTS)
  - Learn coping skills to improve the individual's functioning and quality of life
- What to discuss:
  - How to identify the signs and symptoms of PTS
  - Trauma in a proposed cancer cycle
- Skills to teach:
  - Reactive sets of skills to stay safe and tolerate the moment:
    - Safety assessment and contracting
    - Distract the mind
    - Imagery
    - Soothing through the senses
    - Distract with ACCEPTS and Turning the Mind
    - TIP skills
- Generalize:
  - Create an action plan for a **Safety Contract** (see handout)
  - Create an action plan for a **Skills Implementation Plan** (see handout)
  - Create an action plan for **Experiential Mapping** (see handout)
  - Problem-solve barriers
  - Commit to the individual's plan
  - Review in next session
- Review goal sheet

Trauma and retraumatization

Introduction of the topic

Trauma may be defined as a deeply distressing or disturbing experience. A traumatic response to the diagnosis, treatment, and progression of cancer may be experienced. According to the National Cancer Institute (2013):

Patients have a range of normal reactions when they hear they have cancer. These include:

- Repeated frightening thoughts.
- Being distracted or overexcited.
- Trouble sleeping.
- Feeling detached from oneself or reality.

Patients may also have feelings of shock, fear, helplessness, or horror. These feelings may lead to cancer-related post-traumatic stress (PTS), which is a lot like post-traumatic stress disorder (PTSD). PTSD is a specific group of symptoms that affect many survivors of stressful events. These events usually involve the threat of death or serious injury to oneself or others. People who have survived military combat, natural disasters, violent personal attack (such as rape), or other life-threatening stress may suffer from PTSD. The symptoms for PTS and PTSD are a lot alike, but most cancer patients are able to cope and don't develop full PTSD. The symptoms of cancer-related PTS are not as severe and don't last as long as PTSD. Patients dealing with cancer may have symptoms of post-traumatic stress at any point from diagnosis through treatment, after treatment is complete, or during possible recurrence of the cancer.

Risk factors

The National Cancer Institute (2013) identifies certain risk factors that make it more likely that a patient will have PTS. These include:

- **Cancer that recurs (comes back)** – This has been shown to increase stress symptoms in patients.
- **Breast cancer survival** – Breast cancer survivors who have had more advanced cancer or lengthier surgeries, or a history of trauma or anxiety disorders, are more likely to be diagnosed with PTSD.
- **Childhood cancer survival** – Symptoms of PTS occur more often in those who have had a longer treatment time.
- **Previous trauma**
- **High level of general stress**
- **Genetic factors and biological factors that affect memory and learning**
- **The amount of social support available**
- **Threat to life and body**
- **Having PTSD or other psychological problems before being diagnosed with cancer**
- **The use of avoidance to cope with stress**

Trauma in a proposed cancer cycle

Cancer may not be a one-time event. It can return multiple times over the course of an individual's life, and can even become a chronic (ongoing) illness that never fully goes away. This can create a cycle of potential traumatic events. The cancer cycle may be viewed as three distinct phases. The first phase is the initial diagnosis of the disease, and typically presents the first potential traumatic response. If the individual has any of the previously mentioned vulnerabilities, their risk for developing PTS is heightened. The second phase is when treatment is introduced. Symptoms of cancer-related PTS may be triggered when certain smells, sounds, and sights are linked with chemotherapy or other treatments. Waiting for testing and surgical results can also trigger anxiety and lead to a trauma response, depending on the results. The third phase of the cancer cycle involves facing end-of-life issues or remission. End-of-life issues can trigger a PTS response due to the reality that further treatment will not change the course of the disease. The individual and their entire team of supports may be greatly affected. In the case of remission, there is a common response of hypervigilence and fears that the cancer will return. Any changes in health (either real or perceived) may be viewed through the lens of trauma. This can create an ongoing cycle of anxiety, heightened stress, and misattribution of physical signs and symptoms.

Teaching skills (T)

The sets of suggested skills to teach in this session are designed to increase the individual's functioning by allowing them to effectively cope with trauma and anxiety. The approach and the skill sets proposed in this section are similar to those in the section on Anxiety. There is an imperative difference to note, however, which is the initial focus on assessing for and addressing safety before initiating treatment strategies. Trauma can lead to safety concerns and impulsive behaviors that need to be addressed due to the severity of the distress.

The individual has two tasks to complete: stay safe and don't make it worse. These skills are designed to assist in this process. These sets of suggested skills are designed to reduce high levels of distress and are reactive in nature. They are referred to as "gateway" skills: they can be used to create a path out of high levels of distress where other skills may not be as effective or easily accessible. They are not designed for problem solving and will only work for a short period of time.

The first skill invovles distracting the individual from their distress or diverting their attention. This is somewhat similar to avoidance, which is common for many individuals, but with a distinct difference: avoidance is designed to escape a painful experience and not address what caused the distress, whereas distracting involves taking a break from intense emotions until the individual is emotionally stable and can engage in effective problem solving to target the cause of the distress.

- **Distracting the mind** – Engaging in activities that disrupt current thought patterns. This skill can be used to distract yourself from catastrophizing or ruminating. Examples include engaging in rigorous physical activity, working puzzles, and any activity that requires attention and concentration. Create your own list of activities that involve action of the body and mind. Thought stopping is also suggested as a skill to review in this set.
- **Imagery** – Picturing (in your mind's eye) yourself tolerating the distress. This skill can be very effective if you have excessive worry. Imagine yourself being powerful, like a superhero. Tell a story in which you are able to defeat your distress, focusing on how you are able to accomplish the feat and what powers you use. This can provide information to assist you not only in distracting yourself, but also in devising problem-solving strategies.
- **Soothing through senses** – Engaging the five senses to promote a sense of peace and serenity. This skill in very effective in grounding yourself in your current experience, which serves as protection from rumination and fear.
  - **Vision** – Looking at a peaceful scene or painting. Noticing the visual details of what is being seen.
  - **Taste** – Slowly eating a "comfort food" and noticing how each bite touches the lips, how it feels to chew and swallow. Noticing whether the food is sweet or salty, hard or soft…focusing on the details of the experience.
  - **Touch** – Squeezing stress balls, using lotions, hugging soft blankets. Noticing how the sun or wind feels on the skin.
  - **Smell** – Smelling scented candles, potpourri, or anything you identify as pleasurable. Lavender scents tend to be very effective.

o **Hearing** – Listening to soothing music that mirrors the beating of your heart, such as classical or jazz.

The second sets of skills involves diverting attention: **Distract with ACCEPTS** and **Turning the Mind**.

- **Distract with ACCEPTS** – Accept distress in order to effectively apply distraction skills:
  o Activities – Activities assist in decreasing distress and can create positive emotions. Plan activities and do something each day. Doing something is often better than doing nothing.
  o Contributing – Do something for someone else. Take a break from your own distress by engaging in others' lives in a positive manner. Smiling, volunteering support or assistance, and listening are all examples of this skill.
  o Comparisons – Compare your current situation to a time where you were less skillful and less effective. This can provide perspective to your current situation. You can also compare your situation to someone who has it worse than you do. Validate your experience as you search for healthy perspectives.
  o Emotions – Engage in activities or thoughts that create emotions that are different than the painful ones you are currently experiencing.
  o Push away – Mentally put the distress in a box on a shelf behind a locked door. Take a break from it now, with the intention of addressing it at a safe point in the future.
  o Thoughts – Engage in activities that lead to different thoughts. Read a book or magazine, work a puzzle, or count to 100.
  o Sensations – Stimulate sensations that are safe to engage in.
- **Turning the Mind** – Continually refocusing your attention and concentration away from the distress and toward the distraction activity. This may need to be done continually to be effective.

The last set of skills, **TIP**, is designed to create an intense physiological response in order to counteract the experience of extreme distress (Linehan, 2014).

- Tip the temperature of your face with cold water – Hold your breath and put your face in a bowl of cold water or put ice packs on your eyes and cheeks (hold for 20–30 seconds and keep the water above 50 °F).
- Intense exercise – Calm your body when it is revved up with emotion by engaging in intense exercise for a short period of time.
- Paced breathing – Engage in deep breathing and begin to slow to 5–6 breaths per minute. Breathe out more slowly than you are breathing in.
- Paired muscle relaxation – Continue deep-breathing exercises and begin to slowly tense and relax different muscle groups.

Applying skills and concepts (A)

- Introduce/discuss the homework assignment on creating a **Safety Contract**
- Introduce/discuss the homework assignment on creating a **Skills Implementation Plan**

- Introduce/discuss the homework assignment on **Experiential Mapping**
- Review homework from previous session
- Problem-solve barriers to this process

Generalizing skills and concepts (G)

- Problem-solve barriers to creating a plan for a **Safety Contract**
- Create or modify the individual's **Skills Implementation Plan** to address safety and include the skills mentioned in this session
- Problem-solve barriers to creating a plan for **Experiential Mapping**

Notes to clinicians and individuals

- This session starts with assessing for safety, safety contracting, and reviewing or creating a **Skills Implementation Plan** specifically addressing safety.
- It is important to note that PTS is not a *DSM-V* diagnosis, but is similar to the diagnosis of PTSD. PTS is less severe and does not last as long as PTSD.
- Cancer patients may have a lower risk of PTS if they have good social support, clear information about the stage of their cancer, and an open relationship with their health care providers (National Cancer Institute, 2013).
- An overly simplified cancer cycle was proposed in this section, to highlight the ongoing relationship between trauma and the potential chronic nature of the disease.
- The handout for **Experiential Mapping** can be used for many concerns or targets in therapy. It incorporates thoughts, behaviors, and emotions. Interventions can be applied in each category, as well as between categories. Be creative!

Psychological Curriculum

Psychological Curriculum

Session focus: Increasing resiliency through stress management

TAG
Teach – Apply – Generalize

- The goal of this session is to:
  - Learn coping skills to improve the individual's ability to identify stress and improve coping
- What to discuss:
  - The definition of stress
  - Symptoms of stress
  - Health effects of stress
  - Cancer and stress
- Skills to teach:
  - Observe, Describe, Participate
  - Effectively
  - **Guided Imagery, Progressive Muscle Relaxation, Meditation**, and **Coping with Stress** (see handouts)
- Generalize:
  - Create an action plan for **Coping with Stress** (see handout)
  - Create an action plan for **Meditation** (see handout)
  - Problem-solve
  - Commit to the individual's plan
  - Review in next session
- Review goal sheet

Increasing resiliency through stress management

Introduction of the topic
All individuals have some stress in their lives. This is normal and expected. It is impossible to remove all stress from any individual's life, but there are ways to decrease the negative impact of stress on functioning. The goal is to increase an individual's resiliency – defined as their ability to cope with stress and adversity. When an individual is more resilient, the major negative impacts of stress can be reduced in frequency, intensity, and duration. This can be done through explaining what stress is, identifying what is stressful to the individual, and teaching them the skills to cope more effectively with their stress.

Defining stress
Dr. Richard Lazarus, a prominent stress researcher, defines psychological stress as "a particular relationship between the person and the environment that is appraised by the person as taxing or exceeding his or her resources and endangering his or her well-being" (Lazarus & Folkman, 1984). This implies that different individuals can

have different responses to similar stressors. It also implies that the meaning of an interaction may define whether it is identified as stressful or not.

According to the Centers for Disease Control and Prevention (2003, 2011), stress can hit when one least expects it – before a test, after an accident, during conflict in a relationship. While everyone experiences stress at times, a prolonged bout can affect an individual's health and ability to cope with life. That's why social support and self-care are important: they can help one see one's problems in perspective...and the stressful feelings ease up.

Sometimes, stress can be good. For instance, it can help individuals develop the skills needed to manage potentially threatening situations in life. However, stress can be harmful when it is severe enough to make one feel overwhelmed and out of control.

Strong emotions like fear, sadness, and other symptoms of depression are normal, as long as they are temporary and don't interfere with daily activities. If these emotions last too long or cause other problems, it is a different story.

Symptoms of stress
According to the Centers for Disease Control and Prevention (2003, 2011):

> Physical or emotional tensions are often signs of stress. They can be reactions to a situation that causes you to feel threatened or anxious. Stress can be positive (such as planning your wedding) or negative (such as dealing with the effects of a natural disaster).

- Disbelief and shock
- Tension and irritability
- Fear and anxiety about the future
- Difficulty making decisions
- Being numb to one's feelings
- Loss of interest in normal activities
- Loss of appetite
- Nightmares and recurring thoughts about the event
- Anger
- Increased use of alcohol and drugs
- Sadness and other symptoms of depression
- Feeling powerless
- Crying
- Sleep problems
- Headaches, back pains, and stomach problems
- Trouble concentrating

Health effects of stress
According to Burrows (2006), it is now considered a well-established fact that psychological stress can be a trigger or important factor in a variety of physical symptoms and diseases processes. There is abundant evidence of this link in the medical literature, as well as in current medical practices. For example:

- Medical research suggests that up to 90% of all illness and disease is stress-related, according to the Centers for Disease Control and Prevention (Burrows, 2006).

- Evidence shows chronic stress can lower immunity and make people more susceptible to infections. Conversely, stress-reduction strategies, such as meditation, relaxation, and exercise, have been shown to help reverse this effect (by increasing the number of infection-fighting T cells and feel-good endorphins in the body, for example) and prevent disease.
- Stress has been shown to contribute to the development of heart disease and high blood pressure. As a result, most heart programs incorporate stress management and exercise, and stress reduction now plays a very prominent role in both the treatment and the prevention of cardiovascular diseases.
- Skin doctors have found that many skin conditions, such as hives and eczema, are related to stress.
- Stress is thought to be a common cause of everyday aches, pains, and health problems, such as headaches, backaches, stomachaches, diarrhea, sleep loss, and loss of sex drive. Stress also appears to stimulate appetite and contribute to weight gain.

Stress and cancer

According to the National Cancer Institute (2015a):

> People who have cancer may find the physical, emotional, and social effects of the disease to be stressful. Those who attempt to manage their stress with risky behaviors such as smoking or drinking alcohol or who become more sedentary may have a poorer quality of life after cancer treatment. In contrast, people who are able to use effective coping strategies to deal with stress, such as relaxation and stress management techniques, have been shown to have lower levels of depression, anxiety, and symptoms related to the cancer and its treatment. However, there is no evidence that successful management of psychological stress improves cancer survival.

> Evidence from experimental studies does suggest that psychological stress can affect a tumor's ability to grow and spread. For example, some studies have shown that when mice bearing human tumors were kept confined or isolated from other mice – conditions that increase stress – their tumors were more likely to grow and spread (metastasize). In one set of experiments, tumors transplanted into the mammary fat pads of mice had much higher rates of spread to the lungs and lymph nodes if the mice were chronically stressed than if the mice were not stressed. Studies in mice and in human cancer cells grown in the laboratory have found that the stress hormone norepinephrine, part of the body's fight-or-flight response system, may promote angiogenesis and metastasis.

> Although there is still no strong evidence that stress directly affects cancer outcomes, some data do suggest that patients can develop a sense of helplessness or hopelessness when stress becomes overwhelming. This response is associated with higher rates of death, although the mechanism for this outcome is unclear. It may be that people who feel helpless or hopeless do not seek treatment when they become ill, give up prematurely on or fail to adhere to potentially helpful therapy, engage in risky behaviors such as drug use, or do not maintain a healthy lifestyle, resulting in premature death.

Individuals need to learn effective stress-management techniques in order to improve their health and functioning, as well as their quality of life. There are many approaches that can be effective in reducing stress by increasing resiliency. These include: training in relaxation, meditation, or stress management; counseling or talk therapy; cancer education sessions; social support and skills training in a group setting; medications for depression or anxiety; and exercise.

Teaching skills (T)

The first suggested sets of skills to teach is designed to increase the individual's awareness of what is stressful to them, and whether their current coping strategies are effective.

- **Observe** – Noticing one's experience.
- **Describe** – The process of putting words on one's experience.
- **Participate** – What the individual is doing to cope with the current situation and how present they are in the process.

When these skills are used in combination or in a linear fashion, they provide a process through which to recognize patterns of thoughts and behaviors. They can be used to identify how an individual interprets, reacts, and attempts to cope with an event. This promotes increased awareness of how they typically respond to events.

These skills can also be used to identify the individual's current levels of stress, their triggers for stress, and how they are currently attempting to cope with their stress. Once this is done, they can apply the skill of **Effectively**:

- **Effectively** – Doing what is required to meet needs in a healthy manner.

This skill is important to teach and review when identifying whether an individual's current functioning is optimal or acceptable. Observe, Describe, and Participate provide information about patterns involving stress and current coping efforts. Effectively provides information about how effective the individual is being. If what they are doing meets their needs in a safe and healthy manner, continue the plan. If it does not meet these criteria, however, have the individual select and practice a stress-management technique that they believe may be effective for them.

Observe, Describe, and Participate are also a core component of meditation. Through practice, an individual may benefit from gaining a new perspective on stressful situations, building skills to manage stress, increasing self-awareness, focusing on the present, and reducing negative emotions.

Applying skills and concepts (A)

- Lead and discuss the exercises from the **Guided Imagery, Progressive Muscle Relaxation, Meditation**, and **Coping with Stress** handouts
- Review homework from previous session
- Problem-solve barriers to this process

Generalizing skills and concepts (G)

- Problem-solve barriers to creating an action plan for the implementation of one of: **Guided Imagery, Progressive Muscle Relaxation, Meditation**, and **Coping with Stress**
- Assign homework on the individual's action plan

Notes to clinicians and individuals

- Increasing resiliency is key to stress management. When an individual has the skills and ability to better manage stress, the negative impact of changes in health and functioning are easier to address.
- Caution individuals to avoid comparing their stress levels and reactions to those of others. This is typically done in a negative and ineffective manner.
- Each individual reacts to stress differently: it is not about being "right" or "wrong", it is about finding what works.
- Remember that individuals are doing the best that they can, given their current resources.
- Skills add more "tools" to an individual's "tool belt."
- Interpretations of events are key to understanding the impact of stressful events. How an individual ascribes meaning to their stress can lead them down a path toward either health or distress.
- Remember to focus on effective skills application, take in the beauty that life has to offer, and most importantly – breathe.
- Meditation takes many different forms. Explore activities that can be practiced right in session. Establish a baseline of distress, engage in the activity, and then reassess the individual's distress levels after the intervention.
- Mindfulness can be applied to distressing times, but may be most effective when applied to multiple aspects of the individual's everyday activities.
- Be creative with the approaches in this section: consult with your client about what they are interested in and what they are potentially already practicing.

Session focus: Anger management

TAG
Teach – Apply – Generalize

- The goal of this session is to:
  - Identify signs and symptoms of anger
  - Learn coping skills to improve the individual's functioning in the area of anger management
- What to discuss:
  - Anger as a reaction to cancer
  - Functions of anger
- Skills to teach:
  - **Beliefs about Anger, Managing Conflict** (see handouts)
  - Introduce and review the handout on **Taking a Timeout** (see handout)
  - Imagery, soothing through the senses
  - DEAR MAN, GIVE
- Generalize:
  - Create an action plan for **Beliefs about Anger** and **Managing Conflict**
  - Problem-solve barriers
  - Commit to the individual's plan
  - Review in next session
- Review goal sheet

Anger management

Introduction of the topic

Anger may be defined as a normal emotion that involves a strong uncomfortable and emotional response to a perceived provocation. It does not feel good to experience. Anger is also a response to a perceived trigger or event that requires action. It is a primary target for treatment in over 60% of individuals diagnosed with cancer. It is common for individuals to respond with anger to their diagnosis, their treatment, their medical providers, themselves (anger turned inward, manifesting as depression), and those around them. A person living with cancer may experience anger about the way it has disrupted their life or the way family members and friends have reacted to the diagnosis. Many people wonder, "Why me?", which can lead to feelings of anger and frustration. Additionally, cancer symptoms and treatment-related side effects, such as trouble sleeping, fatigue, pain, and nausea, can make even the most balanced person feel frustrated, irritable, and angry at times. It is important to identify that anger can serve both positive and destructive functions.

Functions of anger

Anger can be viewed as a protective response to a perceived threat. It may help the individual respond to a situation in which their safety is at risk. A useful distinction between positive and negative aspects of anger is the difference between the emotional state that is labeled as "angry" and the negative expression of that angry state, which might be termed "aggression" (Gottman & Levenson, 1992; Novaco, 1983). While anger may serve as an appropriate response to a perceived threat, aggression involves acting on the emotional state of anger when there is a misperception of a threat or when no threat is present. Individuals coping with chronic conditions often respond to situations with misplaced anger or aggression. Examples might include acting on the fear that something will be taken away or that further loss will be experienced (protection), anger responses directed toward an initial loss or change in functioning (being wronged/entitled), adopting an angry style of communication (frustration and entitlement), and using anger responses to meet one's own needs (intimidation).

Effects of anger

Positively, anger can create a sense of power and perceived control in a situation in which these positive, motivating feelings did not previously exist. The perception of perceived control and the feeling of righteousness that can come from anger may serve to motivate an individual and to challenge and change difficult interpersonal and social wrongs. Anger can serve as a respite from feelings of vulnerability, and can provide a way of venting tensions and frustrations. It can supply energy and resolve for use as a defense mechanism.

There are negative effects of anger as well, however. High anger and hostility are associated with an increased risk of coronary heart disease incidence and mortality, hypertension, blood pressure, and other heart-related problems. Anger can create and then reinforce a false sense of entitlement and a feeling of moral superiority. Anger can be used to coerce others through intimidation. Angry people are likely to subscribe to the philosophy that "the end justifies the means."

Teaching skills (T)

The first set of suggested skills to teach in this session is designed to increase the individual's ability to cope with anger. This can be approached in a stepwise and sequential manner.

1. Discuss the functions of anger. How aware is the individual about the roles and functions that anger plays in their lives? Are their responses effective for themselves and others? Are there healthier alternatives to situations that are not working for them or for others?
2. Focus the individual on how anger builds in their lives. Once triggers and patterns are identified, separate the responses into two categories: internal and external. The internal category is reserved for situations where the individual is experiencing potential errors in perception or judgment. The external category is reserved for situations where anger serves as a useful signal that a problem needs to be addressed and resolved.
3. Assign an appropriate worksheet: **Beliefs about Anger, Managing Conflict**, or **Taking a Timeout**.

The second sets of suggested skills to teach is designed to provide self-soothing and relaxation training.

- **Imagery** – Picturing (in your mind's eye) yourself tolerating the distress. This skill can be very effective if you have excessive worry. Imagine yourself being powerful, like a superhero. Tell a story in which you are able to defeat your distress, focusing on how you are able to accomplish the feat and what powers you use. This can provide information to assist you not only in distracting yourself, but also in devising problem-solving strategies.
- **Soothing through senses** – Engaging the five senses to promote a sense of peace and serenity. This skill in very effective in grounding yourself in your current experience, which serves as protection from rumination and fear.
  - **Vision** – Looking at a peaceful scene or painting. Noticing the visual details of what is being seen.
  - **Taste** – Slowly eating a "comfort food" and noticing how each bite touches the lips, how it feels to chew and swallow. Noticing whether the food is sweet or salty, hard or soft…focusing on the details of the experience.
  - **Touch** – Squeezing stress balls, using lotions, hugging soft blankets. Noticing how the sun or wind feels on the skin.
  - **Smell** – Smelling scented candles, potpourri, or anything you identify as pleasurable. Lavender scents tend to be very effective.
  - **Hearing** – Listening to soothing music that mirrors the beating of your heart, such as classical or jazz.
- **Monitored breathing exercises** – Attempting to slow their breathing to the rate of six breaths per minute.
  - Progressive muscle relaxation is another very effective calming technique.
  - Guided imagery is also very effective.

The third sets of suggested skills to teach is designed to assist the individual in more effectively managing conflict. This can be done by preparing the individual for potential conflict (**Managing Conflict** homework) and teaching them the interpersonal effectiveness skills of **DEAR MAN** (DM) and **GIVE** (G).

- **DEAR MAN** (DM):
  - **Describe** – Use Observe and Describe to summarize the situation and identify the facts that support the request or the reason for setting a limit or boundary.
  - **Express** – Share your beliefs or opinions when relevant or required.
  - **Assert** – Ask clearly for what you want or need.
  - **Reward** – Let others know how helping you meet your wants or needs will potentially impact their situation.
  - **Mindful** – Stay focused on your request and avoid leaving the topic.
  - **Act confident** – Use an assertive tone, have confident body language, make eye contact, and stay calm.
  - **Negotiate** – Be willing to compromise to meet your wants or needs.

Psychological Curriculum

To apply the skill set of DM, the individual needs to first prioritize their needs. Make sure that the person they are communicating with has the capability to meet the request. Be sure to ask the right person at the right time. Consider whether it is appropriate to ask for something given the status of the current relationship. It is also important to review whether the request meets short- or long-term wants/needs.

- **GIVE** (G):
  - Gentle – Be respectful in your approach and avoid threats, demands, and attacks.
  - Interested – Listen to the other person and be open to the information they have to provide.
  - Validate – Acknowledge and attempt to understand the other person's perspective.
  - Easy manner – Be political and treat others in a kind and relaxed manner.

To apply the skill set of G, the individual needs to balance the demands their interaction is placing on the relationship with the health of the relationship itself. The relationship may need to be nurtured or repaired before any further requests can be made.

Applying skills and concepts (A)

- Introduce/discuss the homework assignment on **Beliefs about Anger** and **Managing Conflict**
- Introduce the handout on **Taking a Timeout**
- Introduce and review the homework assingment on **Defense Mechanisms and Coping Styles**
- Roleplay anger-triggering scenarios and skills application
- Review homework from previous session
- Problem-solve barriers to this process

Generalizing skills and concepts (G)

- Have individuals share their homework with their support system and professional team
- Problem-solve barriers to effective skills applications

Notes to clinicians and individuals

- Frustration and anger are different – intensity of experience is what differentiates them.
- It is important to review the different functions and effects of anger in order to provide a context for natural responses to stressful events.
- Many individuals may benefit from reviewing a feelings chart, in order to assist in identifying the different levels of anger.
- Explore and challenge the concept that "the end justifies the means."
- Validation and normalization are key to engaging individuals in this process.

- Justification of action can lead to rationalization and lack of motivation for potential change.
- Practice the process of taking a timeout in session, to assist in generalizing the process.
- Learning to take timeouts will promote healthier self-cares, awareness, and communication.
- We all experience anger – it only becomes a serious concern when an individual is angry too frequently, too intensely, and for too long (Novaco, 1985).

Psychological Curriculum

Psychological Curriculum

Session focus: Finding meaning

TAG
Teach – Apply – Generalize

- The goal of this session is to:
  - Learn coping skills to improve the individual's functioning in the areas of finding meaning and increasing hope
- What to discuss:
  - Meaning and distress
  - Physical pain
  - Social pain
  - Psychological pain
  - Spiritual pain
- Skills to teach:
  - Radical Acceptance, Practical Acceptance, Practical Change, Radical Change
  - Just Noticeable Change
- Generalize:
  - Create an action plan for **Finding Meaning and Purpose** (see handout)
  - Create an action plan for **First Steps Toward Change** (see handout)
  - Problem-solve barriers
  - Commit to the individual's plan
  - Review in the next session
- Review goal sheet

Finding meaning

Introduction of the topic

All individuals experience distress at some point in their lives. Distress comes in many different forms and different intensities. When an individual is facing a chronic and potentially life-threatening illness, such as cancer, their lives can change forever. Their reality is altered. Many things that they have taken for granted are now under a microscope of fear, attached to an unknown process with an unacceptable outcome. Health is a priority and can consume all available time, effort, energy, and money. The stressors are real and are faced every day.

Orientation to time is shifted to the present tense. It is common to reflect back on what an individual was able to do in the past and to look at what they are currently losing in relation to functioning and quality of life, and fears of a future that includes distress, misery, and a potentially shortened life. Learning to understand and navigate this process in a healthy manner is difficult, to say the least. One of the key aspects an individual loses is meaning in their existence. Without meaning, individuals experience pain and suffering that has no purpose. Without meaning and purpose, there is no direction in life. A meaningless existence leads to suffering, stagnation, and unanswerable questions such as:

- "Why me?"
- "Why now?"
- "What did I do to deserve this?"
- "Why am I being punished?"
- "What do I do now?"
- "Why can't someone tell me what to do next?"

For the individual asking these types of questions, there are no easy answers. One of the main issues is that they are asking others for answers to questions that only they can answer. They need to discover the answers themselves, through a process of discovery.

There is a form of pain or distress that is termed "existential pain," which can be difficult to define but is mostly used as a metaphor for suffering. Different aspects of suffering may be present in "existential pain," including guilt, painful emotions, loss of a spiritual connection, feeling jaded, losing hope, living with regrets, experiencing marital problems, and feeling that life itself has become painful. Depression, anxiety, and anger are also closely associated with the concept of "existential pain." It is important to explore the role of meaning when we experience a painful existence. If individuals can find meaning and purpose in relation to their pain, they may be able to reduce their suffering and distress. "Existential pain" may be separated into four categories: physical, social, psychological, and spiritual.

Physical pain
Individuals relate first to their physical environment, which includes their bodies. When physical pain is present, it affects functioning and quality of life. Individuals may experience limitations, changes in abilities, financial problems, and increased risk of injuries or illness. These limitations or challenges create a multitude of changes both within and external to the individual (i.e., how they interact with their environment).

Physical pain is a natural part of life that we all experience. It is an indication that damage to our bodies is occurring or has occurred. Pain imposes limitations in physical functioning that tend to change over time. These effects can be either short- or long-term. Understanding that physical pain is a natural and common occurrence can lead toward acceptance. How an individual responds to physical changes can indicate to the clinician whether to target psychoeducation, validation and acceptance, or a change process in order to challenge the potential resistance the individual is experiencing.

Social pain
Humans are social beings. Individuals relate to others in their world, providing context to their existence, gaining a sense of community and connection, and participating in the lives of those around them by belonging. This category includes relationships, cultural issues, socioeconomic issues, race identity, conflict with others, competition issues, and failure.

One of the most distinctive features of this category is the concept of legacy. A legacy may be defined as something transmitted by or received from an ancestor or predecessor. When individuals are faced with their own mortality, it is common to question how they have contributed to the lives of others and how they will be remembered after they have passed. A legacy is the story of someone's life: the things they did, the places they went, the goals they accomplished, their failures, and more. Legacy is something that a person leaves behind to be remembered by. It is a pathway that guides people in decisions about what and what not to do. It's also a way to pass on life experience to others. A legacy leaves behind the story of a person so that they are not forgotten. Leaving behind a legacy gives us comfort in knowing that once we are gone, we will not be erased from the memories of others.

Psychological pain

The psychological category includes how individuals relate to themselves and their own personal sense of identity. Defining who we are, how we live, and our perceived purpose in life is the hallmark of this category. These are some of the biggest issues an individual will ever face in the course of their existence. Thinking about these matters is a natural process for us all. This process can be accelerated when faced with a life-changing illness. Such acceleration brings to light a multitude of dilemmas that can affect all aspects of an individual's development and functioning.

Spiritual pain

This category includes the individual's attitude toward the unknown and how they assign meaning to painful experiences. A sense of connection to something larger than us is a key element. The process of carrying a burden and how we find meaning through it can teach us how to navigate the changes that are experienced. Many individuals experience a polarizing process. On one end of the continuum, individuals can find strength in connecting to something "larger" than themselves and can find comfort through this connection. On the other end, individuals question fairness, wonder why this is happening to them, and find that their beliefs about connectionism and protection have been directly challenged and/or violated. Most individuals shift between polarities at different times and at different stages in their treatment and in the course of their illness. There is little predictive validity regarding how an individual will respond, although there are some indicators. Individuals who find less comfort in their spiritual connection tend to be pessimistic, rely too much on fact when faced with uncertainty, have strained relationships with others, have strong emotional reactions when newly diagnosed, and have many regrets from the past.

Teaching skills (T)

The teaching in this session is designed to be done in two phases. In the first phase, lead a discussion on each category of "existential pain." Explore the meaning and purpose that individuals ascribe to their experience. The homework assignment on **Finding Meaning and Purpose** will help facilitate this process. The goal is to identify how the individual identifies meaning and purpose for each category. Once the discussion has been completed, you can introduce skills training.

The set of suggested skills to teach in this process is designed to assist the individual in accepting their current situation while acting toward change when it is needed or desired. Not accepting reality or changing one's responses to it actually causes one to suffer and creates a barrier to finding purpose and meaning.

Acceptance versus change

Linehan (1997) introduced the concept of dialectics involving a necessary balance of acceptance and change to assist individuals in coping more effectively with difficulties in their lives. Acceptance is the process of acknowledging something without attempting to change it – it is not a matter of quitting or giving up, but rather of recognizing the reality of one's situation. An individual's reality is often an effective starting point for engagement in the therapeutic process. Many individuals do not want to accept their current situation and want everything to change. Conversely, if we accept everything, we will do nothing about our current situation, and we will often suffer as a result. A new set of skills will be introduced to target this key concept in treatment, including: **Practical Acceptance** (PA), **Practical Change** (PC), and **Radical Change** (RC). These skills are designed to assist in the process of guiding the individual through the process of balancing acceptance with promoting healthy change.

There is a healthy balance to be found between acceptance and change. The concept of dialectics may be defined as a commitment to the core conditions of acceptance and change. Progress is made by combining elements that are opposite to one another in order to create a synthesis based in reality. An example would be if I want to be free from distress (a desire for change), but right now I experience pain on a daily basis (acceptance of what is). If an individual is able to synthesize the truth of both extremes, they will have an increased ability to view their experience in a more realistic manner. The synthesis might involve a combination of one or more of the skills outlined in this section.

Acceptance			Change
	----------------------------	----------------------------	----------------------------	
Radical Acceptance	Practical Acceptance	Practical Change	Radical Change

On one end of the dialectic is **Radical Acceptance** (RA). This skill may be defined as accepting reality for what it is. It is letting go of fighting or resisting one's current situation and accepting that attempts to change reality may be futile. It is about accepting 100% of the situation while focusing to change how one copes and adapts to the situation itself. For example, in the physical category, an individual might need to accept that changes in physical functioning are now a part of their everyday life and that their current option is to change how they respond to this reality. This involves a synthesis of accepting the changes that are a part of their reality, which represents a change in their relationship to their physical functioning.

A less extreme version of this skill is **Practical Acceptance** (PA). This may be defined as accepting the situation for what it is, while understanding one can still change aspects of it and how one responds to it. PA is less extreme than RA in that while we still need to accept reality for what it is, we have not exhausted all attempts to influence (change) the internal or external factors that are causing distress. This skill allows for a high degree of acceptance, while encouraging appropriate action designed to promote healthy change. An individual might accept 80% (most aspects that are change-resistant) of their situation while targeting 20% (some aspects that can be influenced) for change. For example, in the social category, an individual might need to accept that distress is limiting their ability to be the kind of friend, partner, or family member that they want to be. They can accept that they now treat others differently, but they still have the power to alter some of the ways in which they interact.

The next skill on the dialectic is **Practical Change** (PC). This may be defined as being able to change many aspects of a situation while still needing to accept that some aspects are change-resistant. PC encourages the individual to focus on action and on changing the situation itself, while also changing how they respond. An individual might target change for 80% (most aspects that can be influenced) of the situation while accepting 20% (some aspects that are change resistant). For example, in the psychological category, an individual might need to change many of their coping strategies to address their distressing emotions while accepting some aspects of their distress that are normal reactions to life-changing events.

The last skill on the dialectic is **Radical Change** (RC). This may be defined as changing all aspects of a situation because no other alternatives are acceptable. This is an extreme skill designed for application in extreme situations. RC is about changing 100% of the situation while focusing on changing on how one copes with and adapts to the situation itself. For example, in the spiritual category, an individual might need to dramatically change how they connect with others or with something "larger" than themselves if their current attempts are causing them to feel isolated, disconnected, and overburdened, and are giving them a sense of not belonging.

The final skill to teach in this session is **Just Noticeable Change** (JNC). This assists the individual in the process of balancing acceptance with change by engaging in a behavior that leads to a change in focus or direction. This is a "baby-steps" skill, providing a first step toward change. It is designed to change the individual's "threshold" of experience. This helps the individual to identify that small steps can have a big impact concerning the process of balancing acceptance with change.

Applying skills and concepts (A)

- Review the individual's treatment plan and prioritize/modify goals and objectives as necessary
- Introduce/discuss the homework assignment on **Finding Meaning and Purpose**
- Introduce/discuss the homework assignment on **First Steps Toward Change**
- Review homework from previous session
- Problem-solve barriers to this process

Applying skills and concepts (A)

- Problem-solve barriers to creating an action plan for **Finding Meaning and Purpose**
- Problem-solve barriers to creating an action plan for **First Steps Toward Change**
- Assign homework on the individual's action plan

Notes to clinicians and individuals

- The topics discussed in this session are emotionally intense.
- There are no "right" answers to many questions. An important point to make is that many of us ask these questions, and finding the answers is potentially a never-ending process.
- Attempts to explore the concept of an individual's legacy can be met with resistance, motivation, fear, and complexity. Involving the individual's support system in the process may be valuable when all participants are ready to respond in a meaningful manner.
- Finding purpose and meaning in life is something that all people struggle with.
- Many individuals may have never explored these concepts, so be prepared to provide examples and be comfortable with not being able to give the answers that are being sought.
- Connecting the individual to respected community leaders, mentors, and spiritual advisors can assist in their journey.
- Be willing to struggle in the process *with* the individual and not *for* them.

Psychological Curriculum

Session focus: Stigma

TAG
Teach – Apply – Generalize

- The goal of this session is to:
  - o Gain insight and understanding into the effects of stigma
  - o Learn coping skills to improve the individual's ability to cope effectively with stigma
- What to discuss:
  - o Myths and cancer
  - o Stigma and cancer
  - o Impact of stigma on the individual
  - o Negative associations
- Skills to teach:
  - o Turning the Mind
  - o Thought stopping and positive self-talk
  - o FAST
  - o GIVE
  - o DEAR MAN
- Generalize:
  - o Create an action plan for **Challenging Stigma** (see handout)
  - o Problem solve
  - o Commit to the individual's plan
  - o Review in next session
- Review goal sheet

Stigma

Introduction of the topic

According to the Centers for Disease Control and Prevention (2011), stigma has been defined as an attribute that is deeply discrediting. This stigmatized trait sets the bearer apart from the rest of society, bringing with it feelings of shame and isolation. It is a common occurrence that when a person with a stigmatized trait is unable to perform an action because of the condition, other people view the person as the problem, rather than the condition. More recent definitions of stigma focus on its results – the prejudice, avoidance, rejection, and discrimination directed at people believed to have an illness, disorder, or other trait perceived to be undesirable. Stigma causes needless suffering, and can potentially lead a person to deny symptoms, delay treatment, isolate from others, and refrain from daily activities. Stigma can exclude people from access to housing, employment, insurance, and appropriate medical care. Thus, stigma can interfere with prevention efforts, and examining and combating stigma is a public health priority.

Myths and cancer

Some form of myth is typically associated with the development and maintenance of stigma. A myth may be defined as a widely held but false belief or idea. Myths are typically composed of two separate but related elements: a "kernel of truth" (some fact that it is founded upon) and fiction. The fictional element can be found when the truth element is overextended or overgeneralized and then loses its connection to truth or reality.

Myths serve a purpose in providing guidance for difficult times and situations. They can give encouragement as individuals struggle to survive life-changing ordeals. Individuals progress in their journey without the education, information, and direction to handle the challenging tasks they will be confronted with. It is important to explore an individual's beliefs and ideas on cancer, since they tend to vary widely across individuals, communities, and cultures. The Union for International Cancer Control (2014) adopted challenging myths about cancer as its campaigning focus for 2013's World Cancer Day. It chose to focus on four globally held myths:

- Cancer is a death sentence
- It is a matter of fate – nothing can be done about it
- It is a disease of the wealthy, of the elderly, and of developed countries
- It is only a health issue

Stigma and cancer

If there is a strong stigma associated with cancer, or if people do not know what healthy behaviors to adopt, they may not engage in practices that reduce their cancer risk. Individuals may delay identification of the disease if fear of stigma creates a barrier to getting cancer-related symptoms checked by a doctor. Once diagnosed, stigma can negatively affect medical decision making, and the provision of supportive care can become a significant source of stress and can increase suffering.

The LiveStrong Foundation recently completed two pilot anti-stigma campaigns in Mexico and South America, which centered on giving cancer survivors a platform to tell their own stories (LiveStrong Foundation, 2015). The impact assessment of the Mexican campaign showed that:

- Three out of four people exposed to the campaign learned something new about cancer
- Three out of four people said they now talked more openly about cancer
- More than two in five people said they changed their behavior in terms of protecting their own health and/or being more supportive to people with cancer because of what they had learned

Results from this campaign indicate that fear and misperceptions are not only deterrents to early diagnosis, but also result in individuals failing to comply with or complete their full course of treatment.

In 2007, the LiveStrong Foundation conducted global research, interviewing more than 4,500 health care providers, cancer survivors, organizational leaders, and community members across 10 countries, to learn more about cancer stigma and how it operates (LiveStrong Foundation, 2015). The results indicate that stigma is pervasive across countries, cultures, and communities. It is characterized by a set of feelings, attitudes, and behaviors that can be compiled into a universal "stigma index," which includes such views as:

- Treatment and support are useless for someone with cancer
- I would feel uncomfortable being friends with someone with cancer
- People can only blame themselves for getting cancer
- I would feel isolated/alone if I received treatment for cancer
- If my spouse had cancer, I would consider leaving him/her
- Cancer is a punishment for some wrongdoing
- Cancer is contagious

Additional results indicate that more than half of American adults (61%) automatically think of death when they hear the word "cancer." Troubling percentages report that it seems like "everything causes cancer" (55%) and that "there are so many recommendations for preventing cancer, it's hard to know which ones to follow" (75%).

Here are some common examples of the stigmas that individuals with chronic conditions experience:

- Distress is a way to escape responsibility (avoidance)
- You are not tough enough (weakness)
- You are not motivated enough (resistant)
- You don't want to be fixed (broken)
- You should…(invalidating)
- You are living off the government (freeloader)
- You are making yourself hurt so you can get drugs (addict)
- You are just a whiner (weakness)
- You are trying to avoid work (lazy)
- You are trying to get attention (needy)
- Your pain is not real – it's all in your head (faking)
- You're really bad off (catastrophizing)
- Your symptoms flare up at convenient times (manipulation)
- Other people are doing better than you are (minimizing)
- What did you do to deserve this? (blaming)

Impact of stigma on the individual
Stigma leads to:

- Inadequate insurance coverage for mental health services
- Fear, mistrust, and violence against people living with mental illness and their families
- Family and friends turning their backs on people with mental illness
- Prejudice and discrimination
- Keeping people from getting good jobs and advancing in the workplace
- Discouraging people from getting help

Negative associations

Another impact that stigma has on the individual is that it can cause them to internalize the messages to which they are exposed. "If one person tells you that you have a tail, laugh and dismiss the message. If five people tell you that you have a tail, say nothing and consider the message. If ten people tell you that you have a tail, you had better turn around." Consider the implications of this saying. If the people telling the individual that they have a tail are all experts at recognizing tails, the message is probably valid and the individual may need to turn around. If the people telling the individual that they have a tail have never seen a tail before, the source of the message needs to be considered. Many people who send messages through stigma may have the best intentions, but they are probably not experts on cancer or chronic conditions. The important point is that if individuals are bombarded by half-truths and untruths, they may question their own experience and start believing in these messages. This is a significant concern that can have a direct impact on the individual's functioning and identity (stopping medications, missing appointments, decreased self-esteem and self-worth).

Teaching skills (T)

The suggested skill sets to teach in this session are designed to increase the individual's ability to cope more effectively with negative messages.

The first is Turning the Mind.

- **Turning the Mind** – Continually refocusing your attention and concentration away from the distress and toward the distraction activity. This may need to be done continually to be effective.

When this skill is applied effectively, it can assist the individual in focusing their attention away from negative messages and toward their own reality and skill use. It may serve as a first line of defense against negative messages.

The second skill set to teach in this session includes thought stopping and positive self-talk (creating new tapes). These skills are designed to interrupt negative thought patterns and replace them with positive ones.

- **Thought stopping** – Say "stop" when you experience automatic negative thoughts (ANTS). This breaks a negative thought cycle *for the moment only*. It may be helpful to imagine a bunch of ants running on the ground like thoughts in your head. This serves as a reminder and a distraction. Then move to the next skill: positive self-talk.
- **Positive self-talk** – Replace negative messages and the "old tapes that play in your head" with positive messages by creating your own "new tapes." Once you have stopped the negative thought cycle, identify positive messages that you can say to yourself. Practice these positive messages over and over. If the negative messages have changed what you think, feel, and do, so too will positive and healthy messages. We have all heard many negative messages throughout our

lives, but we have the choice to replace them with positive ones – and it all starts with you!

The third skill set to teach in this session is **FAST** (F). This set is designed to teach the individual how to have self-respect and self-worth:

- Fair – Be fair to yourself and others.
- Apologies – Do not engage in unneeded apologetic behavior.
- Stick to values – Use your own value system as a guide for your behavior.
- Truthful – Be honest and accountable to yourself and others.

When this skill is applied effectively, the individual can dismiss painful messages by relying on their own values and by treating themselves respectfully. It can also reconnect the individual to their own truth in their experiences. There is no need to apologize for what they are experiencing and know to be true for themselves.

The fourth skill set to teach in this session is **GIVE** (G). This set is designed to teach the individual to build and maintain relationships.

- Gentle – Be respectful in your approach and avoid threats, demands, and attacks.
- Interested – Listen to the other person and be open to the information they have to provide.
- Validate – Acknowledge and attempt to understand the other person's perspective.
- Easy manner – Be political and treat others in a kind and relaxed manner.

This is an important skill set to apply in addressing relationships with themselves and others. The focus of this skill is to have the individual validate their own experience. When this skill is applied effectively, it decreases the need to rely on others for validation, which they may not provide.

The fifth skill set to teach in this session is **DEAR MAN** (DM). Assertiveness training is a key component to setting limits and boundaries or asking for something one wants. The skill set of DM is designed to teach the individual to increase the probability of getting their wants or needs met.

- Describe – Use Observe and Describe to summarize the situation and identify the facts that support the request or the reason for setting a limit or boundary.
- Express – Share your beliefs or opinions when relevant or required.
- Assert – Ask clearly for what you want or need.
- Reward – Let others know how helping you meet your wants or needs will potentially impact their situation.
- Mindful – Stay focused on your request and avoid leaving the topic.
- Act confident – Use an assertive tone, have confident body language, make eye contact, and stay calm.
- Negotiate – Be willing to compromise to meet your wants or needs.

To apply the skill set of DM, the individual needs to first prioritize their needs. Make sure that the person they are communicating with has the capability to meet the request. Be sure to ask the right person at the right time. Consider whether it is appropriate to ask for something given the status of the current relationship. It is also important to review whether the request meets short- or long-term wants/needs.

Applying skills and concepts (A)

- Introduce/discuss the homework assignment on **Challenging Stigma**
- Review homework from previous session
- Problem-solve barriers to this process

Generalizing skills and concepts (G)

- Problem-solve barriers to creating an action plan for **Challenging Stigma**
- Assign homework on the individual's action plan

Notes to clinicians and individuals

- There are extended skill sets to teach and review in this session. This allows for treatment to be customized to the individual's needs.
- Myth tends to be at the root of almost all stigma. Learning to explore and challenge myth can provide a starting point to address stigma.
- Stigma is a daily experience for some individuals.
- Stigma has a direct impact on thoughts, feelings, and behaviors.
- Stigma can reduce motivation and compliance.
- Find ways for individuals to link and apply skills in combinations.
- The lists are designed to facilitate discussion and identify the impact of stigma on each individual.
- Learning to challenge myth and stigma needs to start with validation. Validation (in this case) starts with finding the "kernel of truth," validating why or when this kernel was true to the individual, and challenging its overuse or overgeneralization in order to move toward healthier functioning.

Social Curriculum

Session focus: Intimacy

TAG
Teach – Apply – Generalize

- The goal of this session is to:
  - Gain insight and understanding into an individual's needs/desires in relation to intimacy
  - Learn coping skills to improve functioning in the areas of sexuality and intimacy
- What to discuss:
  - Shifts in roles and responsibilities
  - Added stress
  - Communication barriers
  - Changes in sexual feelings and contact
- Skills to teach:
  - **Intimacy in Relationships** (see handout)
  - **Exploring Roles and Responsibilities** (see handout)
  - GIVE
- Generalize:
  - Complete the homework assignment on **Intimacy in Relationships**
  - Problem-solve barriers
  - Commit to the individual's plan
  - Review in next session
- Review goal sheet

Intimacy

Introduction of the topic

Intimacy may be defined as something of a personal or private nature. When many people think of intimacy, they first think of sexual activity. However, while sexual activity may be personal and private in nature, there is much more to defining intimacy than having a sexual relationship. Intimacy involves having trust in relationships – creating close bonds with others where there is open and honest communication. The presence of shared interests, goals, and activities is also common to intimate relationships. There is a high degree of respect and concern when intimacy is a core component of a relationship. Intimacy refers to both verbal and nonverbal means of connection between individuals.

Issues with mental health and cancer can challenge intimacy in relationships in many ways.

Shifts in roles and responsibilities

Chronic conditions often bring about shifts in roles and responsibilities in families. Many of these changes are in response to a change in physical ability and/or emotional availability. When an individual is no longer able to perform certain functions in their daily lives, intimacy can be threatened. People may respond by being angry, bitter, and resentful. They may perceive the relationship as being unbalanced and unfair. There may be a shift from partner or family member to caregiver. The individual may respond with feelings of guilt and shame, which reduce the emotional connections between people. Finding balance is key to adapting to change in a healthy manner.

It may be important to explore and discuss the multiple roles and responsibilities an individual plays and how a chronic illness forces these roles to change. According to Blevins (1993), there are many roles an individual can take within a system:

- **Blamer** – For the blamer, when things go wrong, someone is to blame. Energy and focus may be spent on the negative consequences, and not necessarily on the individual's responsibility.
- **Cheerleader** – The cheerleader encourages others with great enthusiasm. Individuals typically functioning within this role tend to be positive and popular with others.
- **Distracter** – The distracter draws attention away from problems and toward things that are easier to accept and handle. Those around them may experience a release from responsibility or reality for a brief period of time.
- **Favored son** – The favored son has a special place in the hearts of parental figures or those in authority. They are given positives continually, whether deserved or not.
- **Hero** – The hero finds a way to save the day when things go wrong or people are threatened. They help both people in distress and those around them.
- **Invalid** – The invalid is sick, injured, or otherwise limited in some capacity, sometimes through their own choice. They are often a burden on others, who feel obligated to help them.
- **Jester** – The jester finds humor or levity in most situations. This role helps people avoid emotionally difficult situations.
- **Martyr** – The martyr experiences pain and suffering with little complaint. They are willing to make sacrifices for their beliefs or those around them. A distinctive benefit is the receipt of sympathetic attention from others.
- **Mascot** – The mascot is a good-luck symbol for a family. They are often loved and accepted by others for the positive feelings they give to those around them.
- **Placator** – The placator dissipates conflict between others and can help others resolve their issues. It is common for them to focus on the problems of others in order to distract from their own difficulties.
- **Rebel** – The rebel thinks and functions outside of accepted systems and processes. They are autonomous and free spirits.
- **Saint** – The saint is the epitome of all things good. They are unwavering in their positive approaches to others and to life in general.

- **Scapegoat** – The scapegoat takes blame for things they both have and have not done. They may feel like a martyr, but are not treated in that manner by others.
- **Skeptic** – The skeptic doubts and questions everything and everyone around them. When they do this in a healthy manner, they may find hope when others do not. However, they may also deny the truth when it is present.
- **Star** – The star is given special status and adoration. Limitations are often minimized and strengths are maximized.

It is common for individuals to function within multiple roles at the same time. Difficulties arise within the system when these roles shift in unhealthy or unbalanced ways. It is important to identify the healthy and unhealthy attributes of each role.

Added stress
Coping with chronic conditions can add to the normal challenges of daily life. Unpredictable physical and psychological functioning can lead people to be guarded and wary. This can create an atmosphere of heightened stress. There may be many forms of stress, including financial issues, lack of time for pleasurable activities, and lack of emotional energy. Extra stress also decreases the amount of mental energy that an individual has available. It is important for individuals to learn how to manage their everyday stress in order to be present and available in their relationships.

Communication barriers
Psychological distress and chronic health conditions can affect everyone in the family. Changes may be permanent or short-term in nature, but everyone feels their effects. Many changes may be uncomfortable to discuss – it is often easier and more convenient to avoid talking about them. Family members and support systems do not have all the information they need to be understanding, supportive, or challenging. As a result, they start making assumptions, and healthy communication is interrupted or stopped. It is important for individuals to share their experiences with others in order to build and maintain intimacy in relationships.

Chronic health conditions such as cancer affect privacy for the individual and their family. Professionals involved in the care and treatment of the disease can be quite intrusive. Through assessments, appointments, tests, questionnaires, interviews, procedures, and follow-ups, there are few aspects of the individual that are not shared with the care team. This can be intrusive and exhausting. The individual may feel as if their entire life is under a microscope. They can be left with little time or energy with which to share their experience with their support system. This can strain or break healthy communication. It is important to explore how the individual is attempting to cope with the intrusions on their privacy and the impact they are having on their relationships. It may also be beneficial to discuss those aspects of the disease/treatment that can readily be seen by others – and those that cannot – as the individual learns to cope with their illness.

Changes in sexual feelings and contact
Chronic conditions often affect sexual aspects of relationships. Medication and treatment side effects may cause a decrease in libido or sexual functioning. High levels

of emotional distress may interfere with sexual desire or performance. Changes in physical functioning may cause changes in abilities and increase fears associated with relapses. Sexual contact is an important part of intimate relationships. It does not need to stop – individuals with chronic conditions can still experience pleasure from sexual contact in most instances. Working through any issues can actually bring partners closer together. When people face challenges together, they may experience a new sense of power, resolve, and closeness.

Teaching skills (T)

The suggested teaching method in this session is designed to empower the individual to identify their challenges to intimacy and create an action plan with which to address them in an effective manner.

In a group setting, have each individual review the **Intimacy in Relationships** homework assignment and brainstorm and create a list of skills that may be relevant to their issue(s). They should identify a skill that they could use to increase their sense of intimacy in a relationship of their choosing (e.g., with partners, family members or support systems, or their doctors). They should then undertake their action plan as homework. Have them present a part of the assignment they feel comfortable sharing in the next session. This provides practice for discussing difficult topics and gives each individual a chance to teach a skill they find relevant to their unique situation.

Provide a copy of the **Exploring Roles and Responsibilities** homework to assist in identifying the common roles that individuals have within a system. Identify the primary roles the individual usually adopts and the needs that they meet. Also identify any costs to the individual or their support system that might be minimized or unnoticed. It may be helpful for the individual to take the handout and complete it with members of their support system. This can provide needed insight and opportunities for challenging any fears or beliefs that may be rigid.

One skill set that will be relevant and beneficial is **GIVE** (G). This can assist the individual in connecting with others in a healthy manner. It is designed to teach the individual to build and maintain relationships.

- Gentle – Be respectful in your approach and avoid threats, demands, and attacks.
- Interested – Listen to the other person and be open to the information they have to provide.
- Validate – Acknowledge and attempt to understand the other person's perspective.
- Easy manner – Be political and treat others in a kind and relaxed manner.

Applying skills and concepts (A)

- Complete/discuss the in-session assignment on **Intimacy in Relationships**
- Complete/discuss the in-session assignment on **Exploring Roles and Responsibilities**
- Review homework from previous session
- Problem-solve barriers to this process

Social Curriculum

Generalizing skills and concepts (G)

- Problem-solve barriers to creating an action plan for **Intimacy in Relationships**
- Problem-solve barriers to creating an action plan for **Exploring Roles and Responsibilities**
- Assign homework on the individual's action plan

Notes to clinicians and individuals

- It is important for individuals to address one of the four barriers to intimacy (shifts in roles and responsibilities, added stress, communication barriers, and changes in sexual feelings and contact). It is typical for individuals to struggle with more than one barrier. Start by prioritizing one and then address others in the future, when time permits.
- Intimacy is not created overnight, but is a process that takes time and is built on trust.
- It may be important to discuss taking healthy and calculated risks. "Too much too soon" does not create a stable foundation and does not make up for lost times and opportunities. "Too little too late" is the opposite end of the spectrum and can lead to lost opportunities and relationships.
- Encourage the individual to take time daily to work on intimacy and relationship needs.
- Stigma around sexuality may need to be addressed in the initial discussion section.

Session focus: Problem solving

TAG
Teach – Apply – Generalize

- The goal of this session is to:
  - Increase the individual's problem-solving strategies and their effectiveness
  - Learn skills to cope more effectively in complex situations and with others
- What to discuss:
  - General problem-solving strategies
  - Watching others
  - Trial and error
  - One size fits all
- Skills to teach:
  - SOLVE
  - **Individual-based problem-solving model** (see handout)
  - **Social-based problem-solving model** (see handout)
- Generalize:
  - Create an action plan for problem-solving models
  - Problem solve
  - Commit to the individual's plan
  - Review in next session
- Review goal sheet

Problem solving

Introduction of the topic

Many individuals are never formally taught how to solve a problem. This can lead to frustration, mood reactivity, and social problems. When needs go unmet for an extended period, it is draining on the individual and their support system. This session is designed to assist the individual in learning effective methods of problem solving. Most learning about how to solve problems typically happens in one of three different ways: by watching others, through trial and error, or by applying the "one-size-fits-all" approach.

Watching others

Many individuals learn how to solve problems by watching others. Caregivers such as parents or family members teach certain methods to children regarding how to solve their problems. This is a very common and effective manner of learning. Others "model" certain approaches or behaviors. Typically, a specific process is taught. The learner watches the teacher's approach to the problem in a passive manner. There tends to be an explanation and discussion of the process, the anticipated outcome, and the value that may be influencing the decision. The learner then attempts to repeat this process when they are faced with some form of problem themselves.

Consider an individual who wants to learn (problem = skills deficit) how to ride a bike (solution = skills attainment). The teacher in this scenario might tell the learner how a bike works and about the importance of balancing and pedaling, and might demonstrate how a bike is ridden. The learner is then expected to practice what has been taught by following a specific set of instructions while visualizing how the end product (successful riding) was accomplished. The skill is then learned through practice and a few Band-Aids.

There are distinct positives to this approach to learning. An individual is able to watch others and learn from their successes, as well as their struggles. They have the opportunity to have the teacher coach them through the process from start to finish. They can also see how flexibility and rigidity in approach can either assist them or present barriers. More importantly, they receive opportunities to practice new behaviors, which can lead to new skill attainment and an enhanced ability to generalize what they are learning to multiple situations. One potential difficulty in this process is that the behaviors that are being modeled for the individual may be quite unhealthy. The individual will then repeat patterns of behavior that may solve problems, but also hurt them or others in the process. Think of this process in terms of family narratives. Many family patterns and stories are passed from generation to generation and present as repeated patterns.

Trial and error
Many individuals learn how to solve problems through trial-and-error learning. This is where an individual is faced with a problem, and internally creates a plan designed to solve it. They act on the plan and evaluate the consequences. If the problem is not solved, they attempt to find a new solution, typically by starting from the beginning again. Over time, and through multiple attempts, one solution eventually works and the problem is resolved. This can be a very effective method to apply to solving problems.

Consider an individual who is feeling emotionally vulnerable. A common reaction to this is to find a way to distance oneself from others in order to reduce the probability of being hurt in some manner (strategy). The individual might isolate themselves or push others away by being angry (trial). This can lead to reduced feelings of being vulnerable (success). As a result, however, they have effectively distanced themselves from those who might be able to provide support and understanding (unintended consequence). They have been effective in the immediate moment of reducing their vulnerability, but long-term they have moved further away from needed support and validation (error in generalizability).

There are important positive aspects to this approach. Trial-and-error learning requires the individual to define what a successful resolution will be, since the focus of their work is not the process, but the outcome. A high degree of creativity is needed to identify multiple potential solutions to a problem. The concept of "brainstorming" is often a part of this style of learning and problem solving. A strong work ethic is also an asset to this approach, since the first attempt at solving a problem may not lead to the desired outcome and the individual will need to start over from the beginning. Difficulties can and do occur with this approach. Trial-and-error leaning takes time to apply and may not involve input from others. Some problems require a quick and well-crafted plan. This style of learning does not consistently lend itself well to time-contingent and socially based problems, since the primary goal is the outcome, not the process.

One size fits all

Many individuals learn how to solve problems through a one-size-fits-all approach. If an individual learns one strategy or approach to solving problems that works on the first try, they will often try it again in a different situation. They have been reinforced by having their needs met or having their problem resolved.

Consider an individual who is feeling overwhelmed and has multiple appointments in a single day, along with multiple tasks that need to be addressed. A common approach is to prioritize what needs to be done immediately, and defer things that are not as pressing. Cancelling or rescheduling an appointment may be the easiest thing to do (strategy). This can lead to feeling less overwhelmed (reinforcement). The next time the individual is feeling pressed for time, they might lead with the same strategy, since it worked the first time (emergence of a single pattern). Procrastination is an easy trap to fall into, and the individual may rationalize why they are putting things off in order to assuage their guilt or validate their feelings. This process results in an overused strategy that can lead to diffuse priorities, noncompliance, and avoidance of participation in necessary activities.

It can be helpful to think of intermittent reinforcement. Since a behavior or an approach has been reinforced, it is more likely to be repeated. When it does not work, the individual continually applies it until it does eventually work again. It might be immediately successful, or it might take multiple attempts to gain the desired outcome. The main point is that the individual is not attempting to learn or apply new strategies. "If the only tool I have is a hammer, everything looks like a nail."

Teaching skills (T)

One of the skills to teach in this session is **SOLVE** (SO) (modified from Pederson & Pederson, 2012). The core concept is to use a systemic approach to solving problems. SO is designed to teach an individual to build and maintain relationships.

- **S**tep back and be objective – Stick to the facts: who, what, where, when, how, and why.
- **O**bserve available options – Brainstorm options and determine what is available, but accept the realities of both the problem and the possible solutions.
- **L**imit barriers – Remove barriers that stand between you and a potential solution.
- **V**alues driven – Use your priorities, goals, and values as your compass – pick the solution that best builds your self-respect.
- **E**ffectiveness first – The most effective solution will not always be your preferred solution.

There are two additional suggested skills to teach in this session, which are designed to assist individuals in problem solving in a more effective manner.

Individual-based problem-solving model
The first skill is for the individual who is addressing a problem without the involvement of others. This is done in a series of steps, some of which may need to be repeated and modified throughout the process.

1. Identify the problem
    a. How is this impacting your thoughts, feelings and behaviors?
2. Review your values
    a. Include your strengths and limitations
3. Determine all involved
    a. This includes yourself, others, and your environment (systems you are involved with)
4. Brainstorm potential solutions
    a. Don't throw out any possibility
5. Consider the potential consequences of each decision
    a. Narrow the possibilities and attach potential positive and negative consequences to each
    b. Create a pros and cons list for each potential solution
6. Select and implement the desired course of action
    a. Evaluate whether the plan is working and needs to be continued, or if it is not working as planned and needs to be modified of stopped

Social-based problem-solving model
The second skill is for the individual who is addressing a problem with the involvement of others. This too is done in a series of steps, some of which may need to be repeated and modified throughout the process.

1. Recognize the problem
    a. What is the problem?
    b. Why is it a problem?
    c. Who is involved now and, potentially, in the future?
2. Define the problem
    a. Create your own definition
    b. Consider factors of age, race, gender, values, and power differentials
    c. Get information and perspectives from others
3. Generate potential solutions
    a. Brainstorm potential solutions
    b. Create a pros and cons list for each potential solution
4. Select a potential solution
    a. Consider whether the solution meets short-term, mid-term, or long-term needs
5. Review the process
    a. How did you reach this solution?
    b. Is the "golden rule" involved?
    c. Did you consider all of the relevant factors?
    d. What is your motivation for this decision?

6. Implement and evaluate the solution
    a. Is new information available?
    b. Do you need to continue, modify, or stop the plan?
7. Reflect on the process
    a. What did you learn?
    b. How will this affect others, your environment, and yourself in the future?

Applying skills and concepts (A)

- Introduce/discuss the homework assignments on **Individual-Based Problem Solving** and **Social-Based Problem Solving**
- Review homework from previous session
- Problem-solve barriers to this process

Generalizing skills and concepts (G)

- Problem-solve barriers to creating an action plan for **Individual-Based Problem Solving** and **Social-Based Problem Solving**
- Assign homework on the individual's action plan

Notes to clinicians and individuals

- SOLVE can provide an effective set of skills for addressing everyday problems.
- It can be important to validate that everyone has problems, but the key is to understand what learning style best fits the individual, while exploring the strengths and limitations of each style.
- Have individuals complete the homework assignments for both models – **Individual-Based Problem Solving** and **Social-Based Problem Solving** – for the same problem and discuss the reasons they selected one model over the other.
- It is important for individuals to be taught both models. There are times when one or the other will be more practical or effective.
- Both models address the barriers identified in the discussion section (healthy learning, timing, and generalizability)
- Focus on applying strengths to the anticipated barriers that the individual identifies.
- Problem solving is a skill that needs to be practiced in order to become proficient in it.
- Many skills can be used in both models – encourage creativity in skill use and application.
- Values and morals are key aspects of problem solving. It may be helpful to have individuals complete an inventory on what their values and morals are.

Session focus: Nurturing support systems

TAG
Teach – Apply – Generalize

- The goal of this session is to:
  - Learn coping skills to improve the individual's functioning in the area of nurturing support systems
- What to discuss:
  - Support systems
  - What support is
  - Who is part of an individual's support system
  - Barriers to nurturing support systems
  - Differing needs at different times
- Skills to teach:
  - Building Positive Experience
  - Validation
  - Building Mastery
- Generalize:
  - Create an action plan for **Nurturing Support Systems** (see handout)
  - Problem-solve barriers
  - Commit to the individual's plan
  - Review in next session
- Review goal sheet

Nurturing support systems

Introduction of the topic
Very few individuals feel overappreciated, overvalued, and overcompensated for their hard work and dedication. It is much easier to take positives in life for granted and focus our attention and efforts on what is going "wrong" in the moment. It is human nature to avoid pain or discomfort while working toward minimizing distress. If most of an individual's time, effort, and energy are spent focusing on problems, support systems may feel neglected and taken for granted. This can be a recipe for distance and disaster.

What support is
Support is the act of bravely or quietly enduring something. It is staying with an individual when many others would leave. Support is providing assistance or help. It is engaging with another person and working with them toward a common goal, or completion of a task. Support is promoting the interests or causes of another. It is working with another person on something they find important or valuable. Support is advocating and providing a firm foundation for another person. It is standing up for someone when they cannot do it for themselves. Support is providing motivation

and guidance when someone stumbles or loses their way. Support is caring for another individual even when they find it difficult to care for themselves.

Who is part of an individual's support system

There are many definitions of support systems and they are unique to each individual. Professionals can be a part of a support system. Many professionals work to keep the individual's best interests and potential as a focal point in their interactions. Professionals perform procedures, provide treatment and information, and supply needed objectivity and expertise in times of need. They provide caring, compassion, and support.

Family members can also be a part of a support system. Family members provide love, acceptance, and understanding. They assist with physical, psychological, and emotional needs. They are there when friends would have left. They perform tasks that no one else is capable of or willing to. Family members advocate for individuals to help them with their rights and responsibilities. They share their experiences, hopes, and dreams. They share their fears and insecurities. Family members share their lives.

Friends can also be a part of a support system. Friends provide many of the supports that are common to family members. Friends can assist in daily activities and provide a sense of connection. They can serve as advocates and confidantes. Friends can also provide the objectivity that family members may not be able to, since their relationships tend to be less emotionally involved. Friends are important parts of any support system.

Acquaintances can also be a part of a support system. It may be easier to share information and experiences with people who are not involved in the individual's daily life. They may be able to connect on similar issues and provide a sense of normalcy and connection to "a bigger world." They may be part of a social group or members of a support/therapy group. They provide connection, shared interests, and diversity in experiences.

Barriers to nurturing support systems

There are many barriers to nurturing support systems. This list identifies many common examples and the potential hidden messages in each:

- "I am too busy." (You are not worth the effort.)
- "I never thought of it." (I don't consider your needs to be a priority – I am too focused on myself.)
- "They don't want anything from me" or "I have nothing to offer." (I am not worthy of them.)
- "We fight all the time." (It is easier to avoid the individual or the situation [passive-aggressive].)
- "Our relationship never needed this before." (I want things to be like they were.)
- "I am in too much pain or distress to do this now." (It's not worth the effort.)
- "I can't." (I don't know how.)
- "I can't." (I don't want to.)
- "I won't." (I can do this by myself.)

- "I don't know how." (It is easier to avoid than to learn.)
- "When should I do it?" (It's not convenient for me.)
- "I don't have money to spend on them." (I can only show caring by buying gifts.)
- "I just want to be left alone." (Let me suffer in isolation [martyr].)
- "Things are just fine the way that they are now." ([Denying reality].)

Differing needs at different times

Cancer also presents unique challenges to individuals and family systems. Individuals and systems have different needs at different times. In the early stages of an illness, individuals and families can be in shock, disbelief, and a state of rejection. It may be difficult for all involved to understand and accept what is happening. In times of crisis, family systems tend to be reactive and have extreme emotional responses. Individual responses vary to a wide degree. Some individuals will seek support and information at one time and become quiet and withdrawn at others. It is difficult to predict how an individual or a family system will respond to a life-changing event. It is important to note that most individuals will respond in a manner that has worked for them in the past. Although it is difficult to predict, the best indication may be how an individual or system has responded to similar crises before.

When the initial crisis has passed, a different set of challenges emerges. When there is a degree of stability and predictability present, anger and a sense of loss may be experienced. Unfortunately, it is common for distance within the family to occur. Assistance and support that were given during times of crisis may be withdrawn. Individuals may retreat into isolation and resent those around them. What they were able to do in the past may no longer be real for them now or in the future. Change and the need for change may be forced on everyone. The support system also changes. There is a need to establish a "new normal," as their lives require them to turn their attention to their own needs and activities. If the individual is not able or willing to participate as they have in the past, they may be left behind or replaced, or the system may compensate in some manner. Although some systems can address the changing needs of the individual and accept them for who they are and what they can/cannot do, not all will be able to do so. This is where anger, loss, and resentment may be experienced by all involved.

Once a new normal has been established, all involved can then focus on acceptance and on improving existing relationships and establishing new ones. Accepting that the individual may not return to prediagnosis functioning may be a reality. Healthy individuals and systems respond by adjusting expectations. New relationships form as others are introduced and support systems begin to expand again. The individual may forget to put time, effort, and energy into those who have been with them through the entire process as new relationships form. It is important to focus on balance and maintaining healthy relationships as new ones emerge.

If the disease continues to progress, the individual's needs may change dramatically, as might the needs of their support systems. Physical functioning challenges may result in disability or the inability to engage in previously meaningful activities. The individual may no longer be able to engage in relationships as they have in the past. End-of-life issues and planning may need to be addressed. External and professional supports may be needed to assist in this process. A wide spectrum of challenges and changes may be experienced.

Teaching skills (T)

The suggested skills and concepts to teach in this session are designed to nurture relationships with members of the individual's support system.

The first skill to teach is **Building Positive Experience** (BPE).

- **Building Positive Experience** (BPE) – Creating or engaging in activities that lead to positive moods. Invite others to engage in activities that are pleasurable (e.g., holding hands, playing with children, going for walks). Find ways to spend enjoyable time with others.

This skill is designed to activate behaviors that serve two distinct purposes. It can lead to positive emotions and nurture relationships, which is the primary goal. This promotes healthy activity and leads to increases in positive moods while including others in positive activities. It can also modify activities that have been avoided or stopped due to the impact of physical abilities or psychological distress. The key is to have the individual modify their engagement in the activity instead of not participating in it at all. Modifying activities can also challenge the individual's patterns of all-or-nothing and black-or-white thinking.

A second skill set to teach is **Validation** (V). Individuals and members of support systems often feel invalidated, neglected, and misunderstood. Validation is an effective skill to apply in working toward more connected and healthier relationships.

- **Validation** (V) – To acknowledge, confirm, authenticate, verify, or prove. This concept may be simple to understand, but is very difficult to apply in a consistent and effective manner in relationships.

What validation is:

- Validation is acknowledging others' thoughts, feelings, and experiences. There is no room for judgment, interpretation, rationale, or disbelief.

What validation is not:

- Validation is not telling others what they are thinking, feeling, or experiencing. It is not arguing with others, blaming them, or excusing what you are or are not doing.

One concept to teach or review is the importance of treating oneself and others with kindness. Find ways to acknowledge or thank others for what they do. Do not be afraid to give credit to all involved. Give others compliments randomly throughout the day. Notice the everyday activities of others and participate in them in some way.

Acknowledge past efforts or attempts at support. Recognize the positives in others and take the time to let them know that they are appreciated. It is also important to remember that self-validation is often the starting point for being able to validate others. A little effort can go a long way!

A third skill to teach in this session is Building Mastery.

- **Building Mastery** (BM) – Engaging in activities that have a high probability of success. This allows you to experience a sense of competency and perceived control.

Engaging in BM can be done individually or with others. Many individuals feel out of control or that life is happening to them. As a result they become passive and responsive. Using BM promotes a stance of being proactive and engaging in life's enjoyable activities. This skill provides an avenue for healthy change and the involvement of others.

The last sets of skills to teach are **DEAR MAN** (DM), **GIVE** (G), and **FAST** (F). These skill sets are designed to work toward building healthier relationships. They are most effective when used in combinations with one another. If asking for something or setting limits and boundaries, DM is the prioritized skill, with G and F being used as supportive or ancillary skills. If the situation requires the individual to build or maintain a relationship, G would be the prioritized skill, with DM and F being used as supportive or ancillary skills. If the situation requires the individual to focus on their self-esteem or self-concept, F is the prioritized skill, with DM and G being used as supportive or ancillary skills.

Assertiveness training is a key component to setting limits and boundaries or asking for something the individual wants. The skill set of DM is designed to teach the individual to increase the probability of getting their wants or needs met.

- **D**escribe – Use Observe and Describe to summarize the situation and identify the facts that support the request or the reason for setting a limit or boundary.
- **E**xpress – Share your beliefs or opinions when relevant or required.
- **A**ssert – Ask clearly for what you want or need.
- **R**eward – Let others know how helping you meet your wants or needs will potentially impact their situation.
- **M**indful – Stay focused on your request and avoid leaving the topic.
- **A**ct confident – Use an assertive tone, have confident body language, make eye contact, and stay calm.
- **N**egotiate – Be willing to compromise to meet your wants or needs.

To apply the skill set of DM, the individual needs to first prioritize their needs. Make sure that the person they are communicating with has the capability to meet the request. Be sure to ask the right person at the right time. Consider whether it is appropriate to ask for something given the status of the current relationship. It is also important to review whether the request meets short- or long-term wants/needs.

The skill set of G is designed to teach the individual to build and maintain relationships.

- **G**entle – Be respectful in your approach and avoid threats, demands, and attacks.
- **I**nterested – Listen to the other person and be open to the information they have to provide.
- **V**alidate – Acknowledge and attempt to understand the other person's perspective.
- **E**asy manner – Be political and treat others in a kind and relaxed manner.

This is an important skill set to apply in addressing relationships with oneself and others. The focus of this skill is to have the individual validate their own experience. When it is applied effectively, it decreases the need to rely on others for validation, which they may not provide. It can assist individuals in reducing the impact of conflict in their relationships.

The skill set of F is designed to teach the individual how to have self-respect and self-worth. This can promote a healthier and more positive self-image. As a result, the individual may be less vulnerable to compromising their values and taking a passive role in relationships.

- **F**air – Be fair to yourself and others.
- **A**pologies – Do not engage in unneeded apologetic behavior.
- **S**tick to values – Use your own value system as a guide for your behavior.
- **T**ruthful – Be honest and accountable to yourself and others

Applying skills and concepts (A)

- Introduce/discuss the homework assignment on **Nurturing Support Systems**
- Review homework from previous session
- Problem-solve barriers to this process

Generalizing skills and concepts (G)

- Problem-solve barriers to creating an action plan for **Nurturing Support Systems**
- Assign homework on the individual's action plan

Notes to clinicians and individuals

- We all need support. This is difficult to acknowledge and accept, especially in times of discomfort and distress.
- "The devil is in the details" can be a nice reminder that individuals should recognize and acknowledge the everyday aspects of support.
- Engage in random acts of kindness.
- Remind individuals of times when they may have felt unsupported and discuss ways to minimize the probability of the past repeating itself.
- Identify the positive aspects of feeling validated, understood, and connected to others.

- Remind individuals to treat others as they wish they were treated.
- Resentment and conflict do not provide permission to neglect those who care for us!
- Sometimes the best gift that can be given is time together.
- It can be very effective to pair the skills of BM and BPE to promote active involvement in pleasurable activities with others.
- Not all change is bad – how we react and account for change can lead to either healthy or unhealthy patterns of interaction.
- The reality is that people have different needs at different times.
- While teaching self-advocacy, balance the teaching with relationship-nurturing skills.

Session focus: Managing conflict

TAG
Teach – Apply – Generalize

- The goal of this session is to:
  - Have individuals learn how to manage conflict more effectively
  - Increase effective skill use in relationships
- What to discuss:
  - Conflict resolution
  - Positive consequences of conflict
  - Negative consequences of conflict
  - Healthy solutions
  - Muddying the waters
- Skills to teach:
  - DEAR MAN
  - GIVE
  - FAST
  - MAD
- Generalize:
  - Create an action plan for **Managing Conflict** (see handout)
  - Problem solve
  - Commit to the individual's plan
  - Review in next session
- Review goal sheet

Managing conflict

Introduction of the topic

Learning how to manage conflict in a healthy manner is very difficult for many individuals. Conflict is inevitable; it is not *if* it is going to happen, but *when* it will happen. Individuals argue about many different things, ranging from personality differences to disputes over daily tasks. When individuals are in distress, their frustration tolerance is lowered and many things – both small and large – can become a focal point for disagreement. It is important to be able to disagree in a healthy manner and to manage conflict when it occurs without damaging relationships. Conflict is a part of all relationships and serves many functions, both positive and negative.

Positive consequences of conflict

Not all conflict is "bad." Many positives can come from conflict in a relationship, if it is managed effectively. Without conflict, relationships would be stagnant and there would be no growth or motivation for change. When individuals are open and honest in relationships (which builds trust), they are able to explore how to have differences in a safe way. They can practice accepting others for who they are. They have opportunities to learn from others who think and behave differently than themselves, and become exposed to new ideas and experiences. They can have disagreements and practice building and repairing relationships. Conflicts can deepen understanding, closeness, and respect. There are also times when relationships need to be ended for the health of all involved. This allows for exposure to guilt, grief, distress, and loss. When individuals are able to manage the emotions and the demands of their relationships, their lives tend to be happier and more fulfilling.

Negative consequences of conflict

There are also many negatives that come from conflict in relationships, if it is not managed effectively. Individuals can become very emotional and act from a place of anger. This may break the trust in relationships and can make them aggressive. Conflict can be used to control or intimidate others. Individuals are exposed to intense and painful emotions. This can lead to impulsive behaviors and hurtful comments. Conflict can also be habitual and can slowly erode the value of a relationship, causing it to end. People leave, which can trigger anxiety, fear, guilt/shame, and loss. Individuals can feel unsupported and invalidated. It is common to withdraw out of fear that conflict will happen. Avoiding situations can lead to being distant and emotionally unavailable. Conflict in relationships can lead to neglecting others and the relationship itself. It can also worsen physical and psychological distress.

Healthy solutions

There are three healthy solutions in which individuals can participate in order to strengthen their relationships. These may best be viewed through the lens of scenarios.

The win–win scenario

Most conflicts have multiple potential solutions. The first step to finding a healthy solution involves both parties agreeing that there is in fact a conflict. Define what the conflict is. Once a definition is agreed upon, potential solutions can be brainstormed. The next step is to take the time to explore each person's ideas and potential solutions. This can lead to agreement on a solution that meets the needs of all involved.

The no-lose scenario

When a solution cannot be agreed to by both parties, a different strategy must be tried. This scenario starts with the steps from the win–win scenario. Instead of both parties readily agreeing, however, a compromise is needed. Each party may have to agree to a solution that is less than ideal, but that allows some of their wants/needs to be met.

Balancing the win–lose scenario

There are times when a conflict can only be solved in such a way that one person will get what they want and the other will not. In this scenario, there will be a winner and a loser. It is unfortunate when this happens, but it may be that nothing can be done about it. A healthy solution is to take a balanced approach over time. When one individual gets their way on one occasion, the other should be given preference in the future. When both parties are willing to take turns winning and losing, a balance can be maintained in the relationship. If the scales are tipped too much toward one individual, painful emotions can build within the relationship, which can be very damaging. Be cautious when this scenario occurs frequently. It may mean that the steps used to find alternative solutions were not fully explored.

Muddying the waters
When attempting to resolve conflict, barriers to finding healthy solutions can and do occur. Such barriers need to be identified and accounted for. The focus is on gaining clarity in order to find a solution that is acceptable to all involved. Here is a list of common factors that can "muddy the waters" when seeking a clear resolution:

- Thinking that the other person must lose in order for the individual to get what they need/want
- Being demanding and inflexible
- Blaming others for the conflict
- Bringing up past issues to make a point or hurt the other person
- Leading with high emotionality or intensity
- Bringing other problems into the current situation before a solution has been found
- Focusing too much on what could be lost and not enough on what both parties have to gain
- Failing to gather sufficient information to allow a solution to be agreed upon
- Agreeing too quickly to a proposed solution in order to avoid the process

This is not meant to be an exhaustive list – these are merely discussion points to keep in mind when managing conflict.

Teaching skills (T)

The suggested skills to teach in this session are designed to assist the individual in managing conflict in relationships more effectively.

The first sets of skills to teach are **DEAR MAN** (DM), **GIVE** (G), and **FAST** (F). These skill sets are designed to work toward healthier relationships. They are most effective when used in combinations with one another. If asking for something or setting limits and boundaries, DM is a prioritized skill, with G and F being used as supportive or ancillary skills. If the situation requires the individual to build or maintain a relationship, G would be the prioritized skill, with DM and F being used as supportive or ancillary skills. If the situation requires the individual to focus on their self-esteem or self-concept, F is the prioritized skill, with DM and G being used as supportive or ancillary skills.

Assertiveness training is a key component to setting limits and boundaries or asking for something the individual wants. The skill set of DM is designed to teach the individual to increase the probability of getting their wants or needs met.

- **Describe** – Use Observe and Describe to summarize the situation and identify the facts that support the request or the reason for setting a limit or boundary.
- **Express** – Share your beliefs or opinions when relevant or required.

- **A**ssert – Ask clearly for what you want or need.
- **R**eward – Let others know how helping you meet your wants or needs will potentially impact their situation.
- **M**indful – Stay focused on your request and avoid leaving the topic.
- **A**ct confident – Use an assertive tone, have confident body language, make eye contact, and stay calm.
- **N**egotiate – Be willing to compromise to meet your wants or needs.

To apply the skill set of DM, the individual needs to first prioritize their needs. Make sure that the person they are communicating with has the capability to meet the request. Be sure to ask the right person at the right time. Consider whether it is appropriate to ask for something given the status of the current relationship. It is also important to review whether the request meets short- or long-term wants/needs.

The skill set of G is designed to teach the individual to build and maintain relationships.

- **G**entle – Be respectful in your approach and avoid threats, demands, and attacks.
- **I**nterested – Listen to the other person and be open to the information they have to provide.
- **V**alidate – Acknowledge and attempt to understand the other person's perspective.
- **E**asy manner – Be political and treat others in a kind and relaxed manner.

This is an important skill set to apply in addressing relationships with oneself and others. The focus of this skill is to have the individual validate their own experience. When it is applied effectively, it decreases the need to rely on others for validation, which they may not provide. It can assist individuals in reducing the impact of conflict in their relationships.

The skill set of F is designed to teach the individual how to have self-respect and self-worth. This can promote a healthier and more positive self-image. As a result, the individual may be less vulnerable to compromising their values and taking a passive role in relationships.

- **F**air – Be fair to yourself and others.
- **A**pologies – Do not engage in unneeded apologetic behavior.
- **S**tick to values – Use your own value system as a guide for your behavior.
- **T**ruthful – Be honest and accountable to yourself and others.

Next, the skill set of **MAD** (M) is designed to manage conflict as it occurs. This skill set is similar to taking a timeout and interrupts the process of intense conflict.

- **M**inimize – Acknowledge that conflict is occurring and minimize the chances of acting from a state of anger. Go to a different room or location, let the other person know when you will return to continue working on the issue, and find ways to "cool off."
- **A**ssess – Identify the level of your emotional distress and the intensity of the engagement. Prioritize the skills of DM, G, and F. Create a plan to re-engage

when you and the other person are *both* ready to continue. If the situation is still intense, repeat the first skill until a safe and productive conversation can occur.

- **D**amage control – Do not engage in hurtful words or actions. Do not allow yourself to be hurt or treated in a disrespectful manner. Repeat the two previous skills as needed.

Applying skills and concepts (A)

- Introduce/discuss the homework assignment on **Managing Conflict**
- Review homework from previous session
- Problem-solve barriers to this process

Generalizing skills and concepts (G)

- Problem-solve barriers to creating an action plan for **Managing Conflict**
- Assign homework on the individual's action plan

Notes to clinicians and individuals

- If a more in-depth approach is needed to manage conflict, refer the individual(s) to the Problem Solving section of this manual.
- A key to managing conflict is to first identify and address the emotions that are present.
- Timeouts aren't just for children – use your **MAD** skills.
- Have individuals share their experiences with both the positive and the negative consequences of conflict.
- Many individuals use skills when experiencing conflict, but they may struggle to prioritize which skill will be most effective – *practice, practice, practice.*
- Assist individuals in identifying what triggers conflict and how they immediately respond. This can help to identify where skills can be applied most effectively.
- A balance between DM, G, and F is typically a very effective approach to managing conflict. Leading with the prioritized set of skills can assist the process and guide individuals toward a healthy outcome.

Session focus: Demoralization and remoralization

TAG
Teach – Apply – Generalize

- The goal of this session is to:
  - Encourage the individual to engage in their life in a healthy manner
  - Learn strategies to establish hope
- What to discuss:
  - Demoralization
  - Remoralization
    - Stage 1: Identifying risk factors to effective functioning
    - Stage 2: Finding hope
    - Stage 3: Connecting
- Skills to teach:
  - Building Mastery
  - FAST
  - Mood Momentum
  - Improving the moment
  - Radical Acceptance, Practical Acceptance, Practical Change, Radical Change
  - Just Noticeable Change
- Generalize:
  - Create an action plan for **Remoralization** (see handout)
  - Problem solve
  - Commit to the individual's plan
  - Review in next session
- Review goal sheet

Demoralization and remoralization

Introduction of the topic
When individuals are forced to cope with a life-changing and chronic diseases such as cancer, the process can be exhausting. Not only does it require time, effort, and energy, but it may deplete and exhaust all available resources. This can change an individual's outlook on life. Individuals can become withdrawn, have major shifts in their attitudes toward the lives they are living, and experience reduced expectations of life itself. It is important to discuss the process of demoralization and how the individual can remoralize.

Demoralization
Demoralization, as defined by Frank & Frank (1991), is the state of mind of a person deprived of spirit or courage, disheartened, bewildered, and thrown into disorder or confusion. Demoralization takes place within the context of a past, present, anticipated, or imagined stressful situation. This state of mind commonly occurs in

people who seek psychotherapy, regardless of their diagnostic label. One of the identifying aspects of this state of being is a sense of self-incompetence, and demoralization involves both self-incompetence and symptoms of distress, such as depression, anxiety, resentment, or anger, or combinations thereof (de Figueiredo & Frank, 1982).

Demoralization may be viewed as a syndrome. According to Kissane et al. (2001):

> Hopelessness, loss of meaning, and existential distress are proposed as the core features of the diagnostic category of demoralization syndrome. This syndrome can be differentiated from depression and is recognizable in palliative care settings. It is associated with chronic medical illness, disability, bodily disfigurement, fear of loss of dignity, social isolation, and – where there is a subjective sense of incompetence – feelings of greater dependency on others or the perception of being a burden. Because of the sense of impotence or helplessness, those with the syndrome predictably progress to a desire to die or to commit suicide...Overall, demoralization syndrome has satisfactory face, descriptive, predictive, construct, and divergent validity, suggesting its utility as a diagnostic category in palliative care.

Remoralization

Remoralization may be defined as the instillation of a sense of competency, hope, and connectedness in individuals who are demoralized. Just as an individual does not become demoralized overnight, so remoralization takes some time, effort, and energy. Remoralization may be done in stages, and it is important to engage the individual's support system early and often.

Stage 1: Identifying risk factors to effective functioning

In Stage 1, seven aspects of an individual's functioning capable of tipping the scales toward either demoralization or remoralization can be identified. Finding balance within and between these aspects is necessary in order to promote healthy functioning. If an individual is balanced in an aspect, find ways to reinforce or promote stability. If they are out of balance, promote skill use to move toward effective functioning. Skills to teach in this stage include the acceptance and change skills.

Thoughts

"How do our thoughts get in the way of our doing what needs to be done?" Is the individual engaging in catastrophizing or minimizing thoughts? Challenge thoughts that do not meet needs in a healthy manner. The "I don't know" response can be reframed into two themes. The first is not knowing how to do something. Validate the individual's experience and focus them back on skills they have learned. Identify their strengths, problem solve how these strengths can be applied to the current barrier, and create a plan of action that involves a clear commitment to skill use. The second theme is not wanting to do something. Validation can also be an effective strategy to use in this situation. Validate the feeling of being stuck and not wanting to change things. Give the individual permission to stay stuck, and let them know you will be there to assist them when they are ready to reengage in the change process. Time and patience are key components to this strategy.

Feelings

"How do our feelings get in the way of doing what needs to be done?" Emotions can present as powerful barriers. Emotional distress typically forces the individual to be reactive and, at times, desperate. Safety is always the first priority. Once safety has been addressed, prioritize emotional stability. Individuals typically present with one or two primary emotions that affect their functioning. Assist the individual in prioritizing their emotions. Identify what they are already doing to cope. Separate their efforts into short-term (the next 24 hours) needs and strategies, mid-term (the next 2 weeks) needs and strategies, and long-term (beyond 2 weeks) needs and strategies. Evaluate the effectiveness of their efforts to cope with distress. Modify their existing plan to focus on skills application.

Behaviors

"How do our actions (behaviors) get in the way of doing what needs to be done?" An individual adopts their behavior because it meets needs and has been reinforced, and it may be resistant to change. Problems with behaviors can be separated into two categories. The individual may be engaging in behaviors designed to get what they want instead of what they need. A need is a something an individual requires in order to build and maintain their functioning. It is highly valued. A want or desire is a luxury that can improve the individual's quality of life. Wants and desires seldom have a direct impact on functioning. It is important to identify and separate behaviors into these categories. Once behavioral patterns have emerged, the individual may be ready to explore which behaviors need to be reinforced and which need to be modified. Contingency management is a key concept in this strategy.

Attitudes

"How do our attitudes get in the way of doing what needs to be done?" An individual's attitude has a direct influence on how they approach a situation. Attitudes do change over time, but typically quite slowly. They develop through life experiences, being modified by the individual's interactions with themselves, with others, and with their environment. A key aspect of working with attitudes is to explore whether the individual's current attitude is actually effective for them, for others, and for their environment. Positive attitudes lead to self-empowerment, healthy relationships, and effective interactions within systems (medical, psychological, legal, etc.). Common examples of attitudes include optimism, pessimism, willingness, and willfulness.

- **Optimism** – Interpreting and approaching situations in a positive manner.
- **Pessimism** – Interpreting and approaching situations in a skeptical manner.
- **Willing** – Being quick to act or respond.
- **Willful** – Being intentionally self-willed or stubborn.

Expectations

"How do expectations get in the way of doing what needs to be done?" Expectations can be separated into two categories. The first is what an individual expects of themselves. This is a very important concept to explore. Expecting to be perfect and without fault is a common theme. There is no acceptable option other than success.

There is no room for trying or following a process. It either is or it is not. This does not translate well to reality and daily functioning. The same thing can be seen in individuals who are making positive changes in their lives and begin to fear that they cannot maintain the change. If an individual expects to fail or relapse, they tend to act in ways that make failure their reality. The second category is what the individual perceives to be the expectations of others. If the perception is that others expect them to be perfect in their change process, any deviation from their anticipated path is viewed as failure. They can never live up to the expectations of others. If an individual experiences a positive change in functioning that others have been waiting for, they project their fears on to others and require themselves to be perfect in response. This is a pattern that is designed to fail.

Beliefs

"How do our beliefs get in the way of doing what needs to be done?" All individuals have beliefs, and it is common for beliefs to change over time. This typically happens when something that is accepted as being true is shown to be false due to the emergence of new information. When there is an acceptable amount of proof, the "new" truth is accepted and the "old" truth is rejected. For example, an individual believes that they are not capable of changing. They state that they are too stuck in their ways or too old, or they cite instances in which they do the same thing repeatedly. They make their statements with conviction and believe them to be true. It is very effective to validate that they believe them to be true. If the individual is open to challenge, this can be done through a few simple steps:

1. **Identify the belief** – I am not capable of change.
2. **Identify the extreme stance** – Not capable.
3. **Find the kernel of truth** – Change is a natural part of life, or few things never change.
4. **Identify the challenge** – Change is difficult.
5. **Restate the new belief** – Change is hard for me.

Anticipated outcomes

"How does what we anticipate happening get in the way of doing what needs to be done?" The field of psychology studies human behavior and experience. It is commonly accepted that after decades of study, human behavior cannot be predicted with a high degree of certainty and accuracy. What an individual anticipates as an outcome of their actions has a potentially large impact on their behavior. If the anticipated action does not potentially lead to a favorable result, the individual may choose not to act. The key point is that the future is unpredictable and our actions do not always create a predictable course or path.

Stage 2: Finding hope

Hope may be defined as a feeling of expectation and desire for a certain thing to happen. Demoralization involves disbelief, despair, and discouragement. It can be found in an individual's past (what they have lost), present (how they are now limited), and future (dread of what might occur). Hope can be similarly found. The instillation of hope can provide a path back to a sense of possibility, relief, and restoration. It can provide a chance to learn from the past, explore current options that are difficult to see, and imagine a future that the individual wants to be a part of. Finding hope often requires the individual to have faith that things can and will be different. There are certain steps an individual can take to instill hope back in their lives:

1. Stay safe.
2. Don't make things worse.
3. Do things that promote a sense of competency to challenge self-incompetence.
4. Engage in activities that are safe and pleasurable.
5. When a situation improves, don't analyze first – ride the momentum.

When an individual is engaging in these activities, they are spending less time, effort, and energy in activities that promote demoralization. The result can be the creation of habits that are positive and life-promoting. Skills to teach in this section are the skills designed to instill hope.

Stage 3: Connecting

All individuals experience some degree of distress or pain in their lives. Distress and pain can take many forms, including physical, social, psychological, and spiritual. There is a form of distress or pain that is termed "existential," which can be difficult to define. One definition is that an individual experiences suffering with no clear connection to a known cause. "Existential distress" is mostly used as a metaphor for suffering, but it is also seen as a clinically important factor that may reinforce existing physical pain or even be the primary cause of pain (Strang et al., 2004). Different aspects of suffering may be present in "existential pain," including guilt, painful emotions, loss of a spiritual connection, feeling jaded, losing hope, living with regrets, experiencing marital problems, and feeling that life itself has become painful. Depression, anxiety, and anger are also closely associated with the concept of "existential pain." It is important to explore the role of meaning when we experience a painful existence. If individuals can find meaning and purpose in relation to their pain, they may be able to reduce their suffering and distress. "Existential pain" may be separated into four categories: physical, social, psychological, and spiritual. The most salient point is to have the individual to connect to their experience in order to find meaning. This connection can lead to finding purpose in their distress and pain, which can serve to lead the individual toward more effective functioning. They are not alone!

Physical pain

Individuals relate first to their physical environment, which includes their bodies. When physical pain is present, it affects functioning and quality of life. Individuals may experience limitations, changes in abilities, financial problems, and increased risk of injuries or illness. Pain and distress also reduce the effectiveness of our immune systems, which can lead to increased vulnerability. Connecting to physical distress and pain is designed to increase the individual's understanding of their physical needs and improve their willingness to meet their needs in a healthy manner.

Social pain

Humans are social beings. This category includes relationships, cultural issues, socioeconomic issues, race identity, conflict with others, competition issues, and failure. When distress and pain reduce the individual's participation in relationships, it can lead to isolation, loss of perceived connection, and strained support. Connecting to social supports is designed to increase the individual's understanding of their social needs and improve their willingness to meet their needs in a healthy manner.

Psychological pain

The psychological category includes how individuals relate to themselves and have their own personal sense of identity. Cancer can be a very unique challenge to the psychology of the individual. Identity and how the individual relates to the disease and the diagnosis are key aspects to explore. How they make sense of what is happening to them tends to relate to the "why" questions: Why is this happening to them and why is it happening now? There may be no acceptable answers to these questions, but it is important to address them when they arise.

Spiritual pain

This category includes the individual's attitude toward the unknown and how they assign meaning to experiences. It also includes the individual's sense of connection, which is up to each individual to define. An important point to explore is their connection to something larger than themselves. This does not have to be religious in nature.

Teaching skills (T)

The suggested skills to teach in this session are designed to work toward remoralizing the individual.

Acceptance versus change

There is a need to balance acceptance and change in order to assist individuals in coping more effectively with difficulties in their lives. Acceptance is the process of acknowledging something without attempting to change it. It is not the process of quitting or giving up, but rather of recognizing the reality of a situation. The reality of the individual is often an effective starting point for engagement in the therapeutic process. Many individuals do not want to accept their current situation and want everything to change. This can lead to unrealistic goals and expectations. Conversely, if they accept everything they will do nothing about their current situation and will end up suffering. **Practical Acceptance** (PA), **Practical Change** (PC), and **Radical Change** (RC) will be used to target this key concept. These skills are designed to assist in the process of setting realistic goals and expectations that can guide the individual through the process of balancing acceptance and promoting healthy change.

There is a healthy balance to be found between acceptance and change. The concept of dialectics may be defined as a commitment to the core conditions of acceptance and change. Progress is made by combining elements that are opposite to one another in

Social Curriculum

order to create a synthesis based in reality. An example would be if I want to be free from distress (a desire for change), but right now I experience pain on a daily basis (acceptance of what is). If an individual is able to synthesize the truth of both extremes, they will have an increased ability to view their experience in a more realistic manner. The synthesis might involve a combination of one or more of the skills outlined in this section.

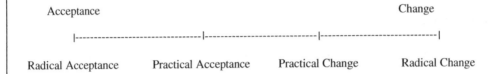

Acceptance   Change

|------------------------------------|------------------------------|------------------------------|

Radical Acceptance   Practical Acceptance   Practical Change   Radical Change

On one end of the dialectic is **Radical Acceptance** (RA). This skill may be defined as accepting reality for what it is. It is letting go of fighting or resisting one's current situation and accepting that attempts to change reality may be futile. It is about accepting 100% of the situation while focusing to change how one copes and adapts to the situation itself. For example, in the physical category, an individual might need to accept that changes in physical functioning are now a part of their everyday life and that their current option is to change how they respond to this reality. This involves a synthesis of accepting the changes that are a part of their reality, which represents a change in their relationship to their physical functioning.

A less extreme version of this skill is **Practical Acceptance** (PA). This may be defined as accepting the situation for what it is, while understanding one can still change aspects of it and how one responds to it. PA is less extreme than RA in that while we still need to accept reality for what it is, we have not exhausted all attempts to influence (change) the internal or external factors that are causing distress. This skill allows for a high degree of acceptance, while encouraging appropriate action designed to promote healthy change. An individual might accept 80% (most aspects that are change-resistant) of their situation while targeting 20% (some aspects that can be influenced) for change. For example, in the social category, an individual might need to accept that distress is limiting their ability to be the kind of friend, partner, or family member that they want to be. They can accept that they now treat others differently, but they still have the power to alter some of the ways in which they interact.

The next skill on the dialectic is **Practical Change** (PC). This may be defined as being able to change many aspects of a situation while still needing to accept that some aspects are change-resistant. PC encourages the individual to focus on action and on changing the situation itself, while also changing how they respond. An individual might target change for 80% (most aspects that can be influenced) of the situation while accepting 20% (some aspects that are change resistant). For example, in the psychological category, an individual might need to change many of their coping strategies to address their distressing emotions while accepting some aspects of their distress that are normal reactions to life-changing events.

The last skill on the dialectic is **Radical Change** (RC). This may be defined as changing all aspects of a situation because no other alternatives are acceptable. This is an extreme skill designed for application in extreme situations. RC is about changing

100% of the situation while focusing on changing on how one copes with and adapts to the situation itself. For example, in the spiritual category, an individual might need to dramatically change how they connect with others or with something "larger" than themselves if their current attempts are causing them to feel isolated, disconnected, and overburdened, and are giving them a sense of not belonging.

Building Mastery, Building Positive Experience, Mood Momentum, and instilling hope
The second set of suggested skills to teach targets replacement strategies for ineffective attempts to cope. The goal is to engage the individual in behaviors that lead to an instillation of hope and guard against demoralization.

- **Building Mastery** (BM) – Engaging in activities that have a high probability of success. This allows you to experience a sense of competency and perceived control.
- **Building Positive Experience** (BPE) – Engaging in activities that improve your quality of life by allowing you to experience a heightened sense of positive emotions. The more time you spend engaging in positive activities, the less time you spend focusing on negative situations.
- **Mood Momentum** (MM) – Noticing and engaging in positive experiences and selecting skills to stay engaged in the activity. It is common to disengage from positive activities in anticipation that "all good things must end." This skill is designed to foster motivation for positive and healthy change.

The third sets of skills to teach are **DEAR MAN** (DM), **GIVE** (G), and **FAST** (F). These are designed to work toward building healthier relationships and connections. They are most effective when used in combination with one another. If the individual is asking for something or setting limits and boundaries, DM is the prioritized skill, with G and F being used as supportive or ancillary skills. If the situation requires the individual to build or maintain a relationship, G is be the prioritized skill, with DM and F being used as supportive or ancillary skills. If the situation requires the individual to focus on their self-esteem or self-concept, F is the prioritized skill, with DM and G being used as supportive or ancillary skills.

Assertiveness training is a key component in setting limits and boundaries or asking for something. The skill set of DM is designed to teach the individual to increase the probability of getting their wants or needs met.

- **D**escribe – Use Observe and Describe to summarize the situation and identify the facts that support the request or the reason for setting a limit or boundary.
- **E**xpress – Share your beliefs or opinions when relevant or required.
- **A**ssert – Ask clearly for what you want or need.
- **R**eward – Let others know how helping you meet your wants or needs will potentially impact their situation.
- **M**indful – Stay focused on your request and avoid leaving the topic.
- **A**ct confident – Use an assertive tone, have confident body language, make eye contact, and stay calm.
- **N**egotiate – Be willing to compromise to meet your wants or needs.

To apply the skill set of DM, the individual needs to first prioritize their needs. Make sure that the person they are communicating with has the capability to meet the request. Be sure to ask the right person at the right time. Consider whether it is appropriate to ask for something given the status of the current relationship. It is also important to review whether the request meets short- or long-term wants/needs.

The skill set of G is designed to teach the individual to build and maintain relationships.

- Gentle – Be respectful in your approach and avoid threats, demands, and attacks.
- Interested – Listen to the other person and be open to the information they have to provide.
- Validate – Acknowledge and attempt to understand the other person's perspective.
- Easy manner – Be political and treat others in a kind and relaxed manner.

This is an important skill to apply in addressing relationships with oneself and others. The focus is on having the individual validate their own experience. When this skill is applied effectively, it decreases the need to rely on others for validation, which they may not provide. G can assist individuals in reducing the impact of conflict in their relationships.

The skill set of F is designed to teach the individual how to have self-respect and self-worth. This can promote a healthier and more positive self-image. As a result, the individual may be less vulnerable to compromising their values and taking a passive role in relationships.

- Fair – Be fair to yourself and others.
- Apologies – Do not engage in unneeded apologetic behavior.
- Stick to values – Use your own value system as a guide for your behavior.
- Truthful – Be honest and accountable to yourself and others.

The final skill to teach in this section is **Just Noticeable Change** (JNC). The **First Steps toward Change** homework assignment targets the work that can be done in Stage 1 of remoralization.

- **Just Noticeable Change** (JNC) – Engaging in a behavior that leads to a change in focus or direction.

This is a "baby-steps" skill, providing a first step toward change. It is designed to change the individual's "threshold" of experience. This helps them identify that small steps can have a big impact on the process of change.

Applying skills and concepts (A)

- Introduce/discuss the homework assignment on **First Steps toward Change**.
- Introduce and review the handout on **Remoralization**.
- Review homework from previous session.
- Problem-solve barriers to this process.

Generalizing skills and concepts (G)

- Problem-solve barriers to creating an action plan for **First Steps toward Change**.
- Assign homework on the individual's action plan.

Notes to clinicians and individuals

- Demoralization is a key aspect to assess for and explore with each individual.
- Assessment measures can be used to formally assess for demoralization. It is important to know whether you want to assess for state or trait aspects, since the different measures assess different aspects of this concept.
- Demoralization is a process that takes time. Remoralization may take even longer, and it may have no definable end, due to the potential chronicity of cancer.
- When promoting change, start small and make sure you can create enough momentum. If momentum can be sustained for a long enough period of time, healthy habits will replace the patterns of functioning that led to the demoralized state.
- Hopelessness, loss of meaning, and existential distress are core features of the diagnostic category of demoralization syndrome.
- This section includes multiple skill sets to teach. Take time to assess the individual's needs before ascribing a set of skills.
- Assessing for safety is a primary consideration when addressing demoralization issues.
- It is natural for individuals to avoid distress and pain. When seeking to reconnect them to their distress, you may find resistance. This is very common. Exploring the pros and cons of their current coping efforts can provide necessary information about when to encourage movement and when to encourage acceptance.

Session focus: Styles of interacting

TAG
Teach – Apply – Generalize

- The goal of this session is to:
  o Identify how pain has impacted the individual's styles of interacting with others
  o Learn coping skills to improve the individual's functioning in the area of social interactions
- What to discuss:
  o Definitions of interaction styles
  o Needs and barriers
- Skills to teach:
  o Active listening
  o **Active Listening** (see handout)
  o Applying effective skill sets (roleplay)
  o **Styles of Interacting** (see handout)
- Generalize:
  o Assign homework on **Styles of Interacting**
  o Problem-solve barriers
  o Commit to the individual's plan
  o Review in next session
- Review goal sheet

Styles of interacting

Introduction of the topic
There are many different styles of social interaction. These styles are influenced by personality traits, situational factors, and needs that have been met. Individuals develop styles of interacting over time. The styles are present because they have met some need and have been reinforced, and therefore have a high probability of being repeated. They represent a pattern of interacting that tends to be habitual. In times of high distress, individuals revert back to styles of interacting that have been "successful" in meeting their needs in the past. These styles may work for the individual, but they may not work for others or even meet the individual's needs in a consistent manner. This session identifies some of the positives and potential problems with each style of interacting. The goal of the session is to identify when the style of interaction an individual is engaging in is not effective, and to create healthier alternatives, while seeking to maintain healthy attempts to engage others.

Examples for discussion
This section provides examples of many different styles of interaction. It is not meant to be exhaustive. It is important to understand that there are many strengths

inherent to each style. The examples are based not upon judgment, but upon observation of patterns of interaction that are designed to meet needs. Difficulties arise when these styles are used in a rigid and inflexible manner. These styles may be very effective for the individual, but they may not work well with others or in social settings.

- **Personalizing** – An individual who overidentifies with the presented information and perceives that others are talking about them or that they are to blame for something.
    - Need being met – The individual feels connected to others and involved in the interaction.
    - Potential social barrier – Others may be annoyed by the individual making the situation about themselves when they are not the focal point of the conversation. It can be a way to dominate interactions.
- **Fixing** – An individual who typically provides solutions to other people's problems even when solutions have not been requested.
    - Need being met – The individual feels valued and productive by helping to fix a problem for someone else. They feel needed and valued.
    - Potential social barrier – Others may view the individual as being invalidating or feeling superior because the solutions are unsolicited.
- **Cheerleading** – An individual who encourages others by being overly optimistic and attempts to provide motivation to others in an unwavering manner.
    - Need being met – The individual feels supportive, helpful, and connected to others.
    - Potential social barrier – Others may view the individual's attempts to connect as being unhelpful, pushy, and overly simplistic.
- **Invalidating** – An individual who fails to connect to another person's experience and challenges or argues about what they "should" be experiencing.
    - Need being met – The individual is attempting to relate to what is happening so they can connect with others.
    - Potential social barrier – Others may feel hurt or misunderstood, causing them to disengage or withdraw.
- **Joining** – An individual who connects with other people through their pain or distress.
    - Need being met – The individual is attempting to connect with others by sharing their experiences with a similar problem.
    - Potential social barrier – Others may feel that the only topics for discussion center on pain and distress. This can also lead to collusion on symptoms and enmeshment.
- **Tangential** – An individual who responds to others by connecting to minimally relevant aspects of the process or content of the interaction.
    - Need being met – The individual is attempting to extend what others are saying, or to change the topic of discussion.
    - Potential social barrier – Others may perceive the individual as not following the conversation or as being uninterested.

- **Competition** – An individual who challenges others by competing with their stories and identifies as being better or worse than others in some aspect of their disclosures.
  - Need being met – The individual can relate to aspects of the conversation and wants to relate their story to others' stories.
  - Potential social barrier – Others may feel offended or devalued.
- **Masking** – An individual who hides or disguises their true experience and typically provides information that is not accurate to their own experience.
  - Need being met – The individual is attempting to appear competent and confident so they are not perceived as being vulnerable.
  - Potential social barrier – Others are not able to connect in a genuine manner.
- **Performing** – An individual who agrees with all feedback and challenges on a superficial level, and then either rejects change or attributes positives/blame to others.
  - Need being met – The individual is able to deflect the focus of attention and avoid real or meaningful change.
  - Potential social barrier – Others perceive the individual as being stubborn or resistant when old behaviors or patterns return once the pressure to conform is removed.
- **Externalizing** – An individual who attributes credit for success or failure to others in a consistent manner.
  - Need being met – The individual is able to give others compliments or to deflect responsibility and blame on to others.
  - Potential social barrier – Others may feel angry, blamed, or disrespected.
- **Help-rejecting complaining** – An individual who identifies a problem and then dismisses all potential solutions.
  - Need being met – The individual is able to avoid changing or "being fixed" by others.
  - Potential social barrier – Others may perceive the individual as whining and as not wanting the help and support that they are offering. A potential unintended message is that the individual is "special" in some way and others will never understand them.
- **Finding extremes** – An individual who uses extremes in language, thoughts, or behaviors.
  - Need being met – The individual is attempting to clarify and simplify their experience by deleting the complexity of the situation or experience.
  - Potential social barrier – Others cannot connect with a "middle ground" or common experience.
- **Emotional sponging** – An individual who adopts the emotions of those around them as their own.
  - Need being met – The individual is attempting to connect with others' experience.
  - Potential social barrier – The individual overconnects with others and experiences emotions out of context to their own lives. Responsibility for emotions and overall experience becomes diffuse.

Teaching skills (T)

The teaching in this session is designed to be interactive through roleplaying active listening skills. The suggested sets of skills to teach are **Active Listening** skills (see handout). These skills can provide a foundation for healthy communication.

Applying skills and concepts (A)

- Introduce/discuss the homework assignment on **Styles of Interacting**
- Roleplay active listening skills using the **Active Listening** handout
- Review homework from the previous session
- Problem-solve barriers to this process

Generalizing skills and concepts (G)

- Problem-solve barriers to creating an action plan for **Styles of Interacting**
- Assign homework on the individual's action plan

Notes to clinicians and individuals

- Styles of interaction are neither "good" nor "bad" and we all behave in certain ways. It is important to identify when interaction styles are ineffective and find healthier alternatives.
- Individuals may need to consult those around them to assist in identifying patterns of interaction. This is due to a lack of insight into their own styles. Gathering information from others may be helpful in identifying what is working and what is not.
- It may be important to assess whether needs are being met in the short, medium, and long term. Often, needs are met in the short term, but there is actually a negative impact on relationships when a pattern of interacting is repeated over time.
- Challenging judgment can assist individuals in being open to feedback and willing to change.
- Many individuals are able to adopt different styles of interacting. When high degrees of distress are present, it is common to regress to a singular or limited approach to interacting with others. This can limit functioning and social connectedness.
- Finding a balance of what works for the individual and others is a primary goal of this session.

Session focus: Grief and loss

TAG
Teach – Apply – Generalize

- The goal of this session is to:
  - Learn coping skills to improve the individual's ability to cope effectively in the areas of daily grief and loss
- What to discuss:
  - Grief
  - Loss:
    - Identity
    - Insecurity
    - Isolation
- Skills to teach:
  - DEAR MAN
  - FAST
  - Wise Mind
  - Opposite to Emotion
- Generalize:
  - Create an action plan for **The 3 I's**
  - Problem-solve barriers
  - Commit to the individual's plan
  - Review in next session
- Review goal sheet

Grief and loss

Introduction of the topic
Cancer can affect all aspects of an individual's life. There is no way to knowingly predict an individual's response to the initial diagnosis or their responses throughout the course of the disease itself. Since cancer is a disease that may be chronic in nature, the one thing that can be predicted is change. Change is inevitable. With change comes a sense of grief and loss, which is a common experience for individuals diagnosed with cancer.

Grief
A common definition of grief is deep and poignant distress, typically associated with bereavement. Grief does not require the loss of a loved one, but can be and is experienced by many individuals diagnosed with cancer. It is important to understand the many aspects of grief, which include: "sorrow, misery, sadness, anguish, pain, distress, heartache, heartbreak, agony, torment, affliction, suffering, woe, desolation, dejection, and despair" (Colbert, 2013). Although this is not an exhaustive list, it is an understatement to say that grief is a complicated state of emotions and experiences.

Elisabeth Kübler-Ross (1969) identified five stages of grief. This model can be a helpful discussion topic in therapy. Although her initial intent was not to present a stage-model of the grief process, this presentation of her work has become common use in therapy:

- **Denial** – The individual denies the reality of being diagnosed with an unacceptable condition. This is a deflection response, used to deal with the shock and distress they are experiencing.
- **Anger** – When the individual recognizes that denial cannot continue, their pain and distress re-emerge. They become frustrated and angry due to feeling vulnerable. Targets for these intense emotions can range from inanimate objects to the professionals involved in their care.
- **Bargaining** – This is where the individual hopes they can avoid the cause of their distress. This usually involves some form of attempted negotiation to gain health and control by offering some form of attempted reform.
- **Depression** – Sadness and regret are common responses when the individual's attempts to cope are not effective. This may be a short-term response, but it may also be present for an extended period of time.
- **Acceptance** – Facing the reality of the situation can lead to a sense of calm and emotional stability.

An individual's needs and how they access their social supports will change as they go through the grieving process. There are times where emotional stability is a priority, and other times when connecting with others is the most pressing need. There is a high degree of unpredictability attached to this process and the presented model outlines commonalities.

Loss
Experiencing loss is common to any change process. When the change is initiated and guided by the individual, the perception of loss is more easily rationalized and accepted. When change is forced on the individual, a sense of loss may be a part of their primary experience. Typical losses include changes in identity, maintaining a sense of security, and becoming distanced from supports. These concepts may be referred to as the "3 I's" for the sake of discussion.

Identity
Identity may be defined as the unique features or personality of an individual. This means that all individuals are unique and have distinct differences from other people. A diagnosis of cancer can challenge an individual's identity. They become labeled as a "patient" or "consumer." They are referred to by their symptoms, treatment, and stage progression, or labeled as a "survivor." Labels serve the function of conveying a lot of information quickly. They are used frequently when individuals are working with insurance companies and professionals. It is also common to experience these labels through media or when accessing community supports, such as support groups. Labels and classifications present challenges. They may make the individual feel like they are their illness. The individual may feel like they are being talked at and about instead of

being talked to. Labels also dehumanize the individual. They are no longer referred to by name first, but through their relation to their illness or disease. Individuals can feel disconnected from their teams and supports. Many individuals may feel like things are happening to them and they are not involved in making decisions with others. These examples can all challenge an individual's sense of identity.

Insecurity

When an individual is first diagnosed with cancer, they are thrust into a new world. They need to learn new terms, understand new treatments, and explore available options. Their world is forced to change rapidly. There are many new experiences that are novel and threatening. Insecurity is a natural response when feeling threatened, unsure, and afraid. Many individuals will seek to access their support systems of professionals and personal supports, such as family, friends, and groups of people faced with similar challenges. This can become problematic when their requests for support are too taxing on the systems. The individual may not be ready or know how to access available supports. They may make many phone calls to professionals in an attempt to get some of their questions answered. Professionals tend to be busy and may not be able to return calls in a timely manner. When contact is made, the calls may be rushed or there may not be "good" or acceptable answers to all of the questions. Repeated attempts may lead to labels such as "problematic patient" or "difficult client." This situation can make fears worse. Searching the Internet for answers can also lead to problems. There is a lot of information available that may not be relevant to the individual, or even accurate to their situation. Individuals may respond by overidentifying with misinformation, symptoms, treatments, and possible outcomes. This can lead to anger, isolation, and despair. Personal support systems can also be threatened. Individuals may become too "needy" or "clingy" when seeking support or reassurance. They may feel guilt and shame as a result and respond by intensifying their attempts to gain support, or they may withdraw and feel rejected and unloved.

Isolation

Feelings of fear, insecurity, and rejection commonly lead to the urge for isolation. When individuals do not feel understood, supported, or connected, they tend to withdraw from others. It is important to separate urges from action. Individuals may have the urge to isolate, but the state of isolation is attained through the action of withdrawing. Isolation is a protective state of being for many individuals. It may feel safer to be in isolation than to be around others. This can become problematic when the act of withdrawing is reinforced and becomes habit. If an individual feels threatened in some way, has an urge to isolate, acts on the urge, and feels safer by avoiding the threatening situation, they are more apt to repeat this process. Being in the state of isolation may feel safer for a short period of time, but like other avoidance strategies there are many negatives attached to this coping strategy. Being in the state of isolation can lead to catastrophizing, rumination on fears, becoming disconnected from others, failure to access needed supports and services, and worsening of other symptoms of depression and anxiety. The state of isolation can be viewed as practicing the symptoms of distress.

Teaching skills (T)

The suggested skills to teach in this session are designed to assist the individual in coping more effectively with grief, identity, insecurity, and isolation.

Assertiveness training is a key component to setting limits and boundaries or asking for something the individual wants. As they navigate the grieving process, it is expected that their needs, wants, and desires will change. It is important to address the level of intensity that is needed when using this skill. Higher levels of intensity may be needed when addressing a need, and lower levels when addressing a want. The skill set of **DEAR MAN** (DM) is designed to teach the individual to increase the probability of getting their wants or needs met.

- **D**escribe – Use Observe and Describe to summarize the situation and identify the facts that support the request or the reason for setting a limit or boundary.
- **E**xpress – Share your beliefs or opinions when relevant or required.
- **A**ssert – Ask clearly for what you want or need.
- **R**eward – Let others know how helping you meet your wants or needs will potentially impact their situation.
- **M**indful – Stay focused on your request and avoid leaving the topic.
- **A**ct confident – Use an assertive tone, have confident body language, make eye contact, and stay calm.
- **N**egotiate – Be willing to compromise to meet your wants or needs.

The second skill set to teach in this session may be applied to working with the individual's identity. The skill set of **FAST** (F) is designed to teach the individual how to have self-respect and self-worth. This can promote a healthier and more positive self-image. As a result, the individual may be less vulnerable to threats to their identity.

- **F**air – Be fair to yourself and others.
- **A**pologies – Do not engage in unneeded apologetic behavior.
- **S**tick to values – Use your own value system as a guide for your behavior.
- **T**ruthful – Be honest and accountable to yourself and others.

It is important to have individuals act through their existing roles in order to challenge the impact of labeling. Act as a mother/father or son/daughter, and challenge labels when they are experienced. Identify the current values that are relevant to the situation and use language and actions that represent those values. This humanizes the situation and provides challenges to labeling and stigma. If an individual behaves like an individual, they increase the probability that others will treat them accordingly.

The concept of **Wise Mind** (WM) can be used to find balance between feelings of security and insecurity. It represents a balance between emotion and reason. Individuals experience three primary states of mind, which all have different strengths and vulnerabilities: Emotion Mind, Reason Mind, and Wise Mind. It is easier to explain these concepts when they are placed on a continuum.

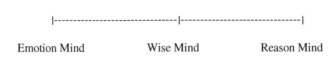

|------------------------------|------------------------------|

Emotion Mind   Wise Mind   Reason Mind

- **Emotion Mind** – The state of mind in which emotions are the primary influence on thoughts and behaviors. This represents a state of imbalance in which individuals may be very creative, but are also highly impulsive and reactive. When individuals are feeling insecure, they are emotionally reactive and not thinking clearly.
- **Reason Mind** – The state of mind in which an individual is logical, thinking, and rational. This represents a state of imbalance in which individuals can be "cool, planful, and calculating," but are also quite distanced from their emotions and may not be aware of how their emotions are influencing them. When individuals are feeling insecure, moving into Reason Mind may provide initial distance from painful emotions, but can also lead to catastrophizing and rumination.
- **Wise Mind** – The state of mind in which emotions and thoughts are balanced. This represents a healthy combination of thinking and feeling, which is a goal-state for therapy. When individuals are feeling insecure, finding balance allows them to validate their own experience and select behaviors with a higher probability of meeting their needs in an effective manner.

The last set of skills, **Opposite to Emotion** (O2E), is designed to assist the individual in coping more effectively with urges to isolate. The goal is to be able to identify the urge to isolate, and replace the behavior of withdrawing with behaviors that promote connection with others.

- **Opposite to Emotion** (O2E) – Use opposite actions to avoid negative emotions. If you experience the urge to isolate, engage in activities that connect you to others.

By acting opposite to their urge to isolate, the individual will not only change their behaviors, but will typically change the outcome and not end in isolation. Have them create a list of possible actions that will assist them in connecting with their support systems. Applying the skill of O2E interrupts the isolation cycle and replaces withdrawal behaviors with healthier actions.

Applying skills and concepts (A)

- Introduce/discuss the homework assignment on **The 3 I's**
- Review homework from previous session
- Problem-solve barriers to this process

Generalizing skills and concepts (G)

- Problem-solve barriers to creating an action plan for **The 3 I's**
- Assign homework on the individual's action plan

Notes to clinicians and individuals

- The stages of grief model by Kübler-Ross is important to discuss. It can provide needed information about the process and role that grief is playing in the individual's life.
- When using the DM skill, it is easier to start with a lower level of intensity and raise it if needed. It is much more difficult to start with high intensity and then lower it as the situation changes.
- Social responses to cancer vary widely!
- It is expected that many individuals will struggle with all three of the issues presented in this session. Prioritize the needs and address them in order.
- Multiple skill sets are relevant to the work in this session. Review other sessions to select skills that may be relevant to the individual.
- Finding balance is quite difficult, but can be accomplished through consistent skill use and awareness.
- You are not your disease.
- There is never an instance in which nothing can be done.

Handouts and Homework

CBT for Psychological Well-Being in Cancer: A Skills Training Manual Integrating DBT, ACT, Behavioral Activation and Motivational Interviewing, First Edition. Mark Carlson.
© 2017 John Wiley & Sons, Ltd. Published 2017 by John Wiley & Sons, Ltd.

General Curriculum

Group Rules/Expectations

Group members are expected to attend each scheduled session. Absences must be planned with the therapist and/or group in advance. Documentation of absences may be requested. Attendance below 85% will result in an attendance contract. Three consecutive absences without phone calls will be grounds for discharge.

- Members must maintain confidentiality. Group issues cannot be discussed outside of group or during break. Breaking confidentiality may be grounds for discharge.
- Members are expected to participate in group through active listening, providing support and feedback to peers, being engaged in teaching, presenting tracking cards, and completing behavior/cognitive analysis and homework, as assigned.
- Members are expected to take problem solving time and practice skills whenever they report significant distress.
- Members' feedback and behavior is expected to be respectful at all times. Anyone engaged in disrespectful feedback will be given a verbal warning and then may be asked to take a break or leave. Examples of disrespectful behavior include:
  o Interrupting others
  o Using inappropriate verbal and/or nonverbal language
  o Sharing specific details of behaviors that are self-injurious
  o Not respecting the boundaries of others
  A pattern of disrespectful behavior may result in a behavior contract, suspension, or discharge from group.
- Members are encouraged to use one another for support outside of group. However, members are expected to be clear and respectful of one another's boundaries. Members are not allowed to have romantic or other private relationships with one another.
- Members are not allowed to use alcohol or drugs, or to engage in unhealthy behaviors together. Participating in these behaviors may be grounds for discharge.
- Members are not allowed to engage in SI/SIB behaviors on the premises or to come to group under the influence of alcohol or drugs. Such behaviors may be grounds for discharge.
- Members may not call other members for 24 hours after they have acted on SI/SIB/TIB behaviors.
- Members are required to participate in ongoing individual therapy and comply with prescribed medications.
- Members are expected to comply with their payment agreements.

Acknowledged by: _____

NAME: _____

Attendance/Discharge Contract

- Because your attendance is below 85%, you will go on an attendance or discharge contract. Note that an attendance contract precedes a discharge contract.
- Attendance and discharge contracts require you to attend at least 5 out of the next 6 sessions (85%), starting the day of the contract (you get credit for today if you are in program).
- When you successfully complete either an attendance or a discharge contract, it automatically ends.
- If you miss more than 1 time during the attendance contract, you will go on a discharge contract.
- If you miss more than 1 time during the discharge contract, you will be discharged from group at the time of your second absence.
- If discharged, you cannot reapply to group for 3 months.

Please note: Attendance and discharge contracts are intended to help you to stay committed to the program and your own goals and recovery. Use this as an opportunity to talk with your therapist and team members about issues that need to be addressed in order to increase your success.

Date of **attendance/discharge** (*circle one*) contract: _____

Treatment team contacted: yes/no (*circle one*)

Acknowledged by:

_____   Date: _____
Client

_____   Date: _____
Therapist

NAME: _____

Safety Contract

I, _____, contract for my safety. This means I will not act on my plan to commit suicide. I will use the skills listed below to assist with my safety, call my team members/people in my support system/crisis numbers listed below as needed, or admit myself into the hospital if needed. I agree to follow these steps BEFORE I act on urges on purpose or by accident.

Skills/other activities I will use to maintain my safety:

1.
2.
3.
4.
5.

Team members/other people in my support system/crisis numbers I can call for help are:

1. Phone number:
2. Phone number:
3. Phone number:
4. Crisis Connection
5. National Suicide Prevention Lifeline 1-800-273-8255
6. Emergency 911

Acknowledged by:

_____ Date: _____
Client

_____ Date: _____
Therapist

NAME: _____

Skills Implementation Plan

Crisis Behavior: _____

List below behaviors, feelings, and situations typically associated with the crisis at each scale level.

0 NO CRISIS
List typical situation: _____
List typical thoughts: _____
　　　　feelings: _____
　　　　behaviors: _____
Skills to use: _____

1–2 EARLY WARNING SIGNS
List typical situation: _____
List typical thoughts: _____
　　　　feelings: _____
　　　　behaviors: _____
Skills to use: _____

3–4 SOME DISTRESS
List typical situation: _____
List typical thoughts: _____
　　　　feelings: _____
　　　　behaviors: _____
Skills to use: _____

5–6 INCREASED DISTRESS
List typical situation: _____
List typical thoughts: _____
　　　　feelings: _____
　　　　behaviors: _____
Skills to use: _____

7–8 INTENSE DISTRESS
List typical situation: _____
List typical thoughts: _____
　　　　feelings: _____
　　　　behaviors: _____
Skills to use: _____

9–10 CRISIS POINT
List typical situation: _____
List typical thoughts: _____
　　　　feelings: _____
　　　　behaviors: _____

Skills to use: _____

DIAGNOSES	SYMPTOMS

MEDICATIONS

1. _____   Dosage _____
2. _____   Dosage _____
3. _____   Dosage _____
4. _____   Dosage _____
5. _____   Dosage _____
6. _____   Dosage _____
7. _____   Dosage _____

MEDICAL ALERTS _____

CONTACTS

List people (friends and mental health team members) to call for support in the event of crisis):

Therapist: _____   Phone # _____
Psychiatrist: _____   Phone # _____
Case manager: _____   Phone # _____
Friend: _____   Phone # _____
Other: _____   Phone # _____
Other: _____   Phone # _____

(Adapted from Pederson & Pederson, 2012)

Cognitive Mapping

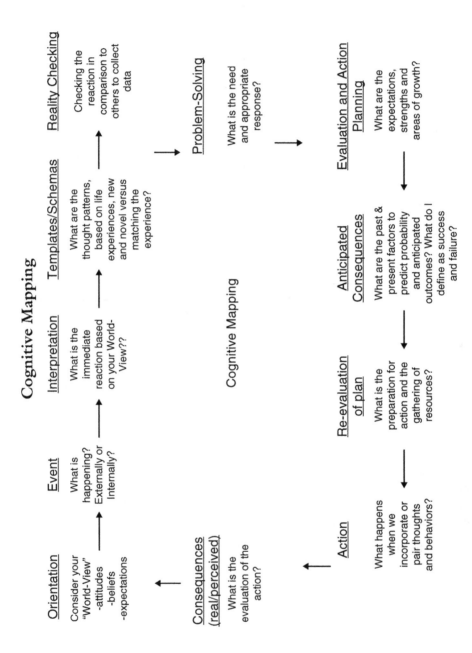

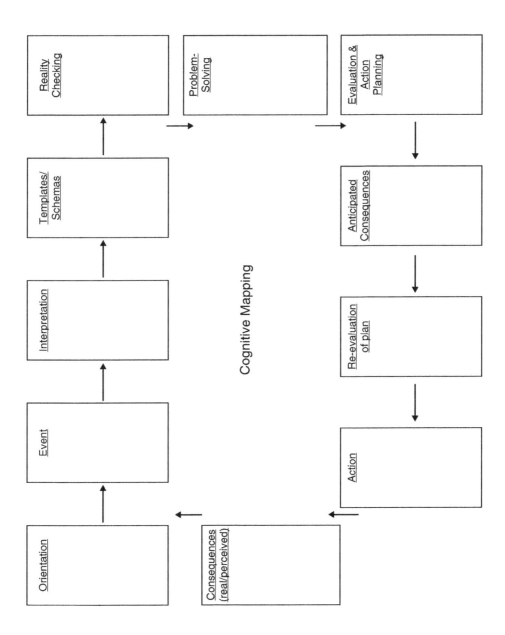

Cognitive Mapping

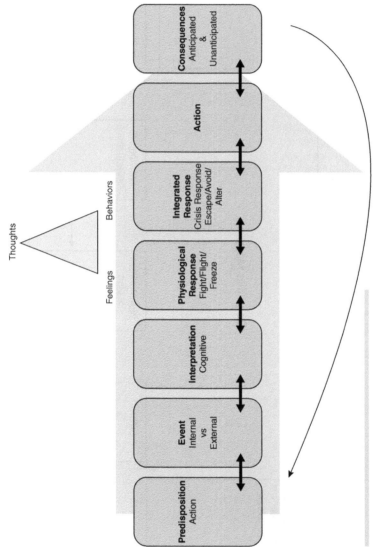

Behavioral Mapping

Thoughts

Behaviors

Feelings

Predisposition	Event	Interpretation	Physiological Response	Integrated Response	Action	Consequences
Action	Internal vs External	Cognitive	Fight/Flight/ Freeze	Crisis Response Escape/Avoid/ Alter		Anticipated & Unanticipated

Time—slow things down for insight and options
Process—overall process for insight
Psychology of progression—can cycle between
Intensity—increased if needs do not get met
Behavior—pattern recognition

Goal Setting

Vision of Recovery (VOR)

An individual's VOR is the first step in setting realistic goals. The VOR is the "bigger picture" for the individual. This is where the individual identifies what they would want their lives to look like if they no longer needed consistent medical and mental health services at their current level of intensity.

This is one of the first opportunities for the individual to identify their hopes and dreams. It provides an initial direction for therapy. It may also identify strengths and motivation to work toward positive change in their lives. Here are a few examples of questions the clinician can pose to the individual:

- What do you want your life to look like in the next few years?
- What do you want out of life?
- What do you want your life to look like when you are no longer in primary treatment?
- Can you imagine what your life will look like when you are no longer in treatment?
- What do you want your life to look like when pain or illness is no longer controlling it?

Goals

Once the VOR has been established, it is time to begin working on defining the individual's goals. Goals can be viewed as the degree and direction in which an individual needs to work in order to move closer to their VOR. This is the first step in operationally defining an individual's treatment. Specific targets are identified for treatment that reduces the individual's ability to cope effectively or to function at a higher level. Timelines are typically attached to goals in order to establish review periods in which to assess movement throughout the therapeutic process. This is the "middle ground" between the VOR and the specific steps to beginning work. It is important to incorporate the individual's own words in order to promote ownership in the process. If the clinician does not incorporate the individual in the creation process, this will allow for externalization, decreased motivation, and less perceived control, all of which lead to demoralization and decreased hope. Perceived power and control are necessary ingredients in the promotion and reinforcement of motivation. Here are a few examples of questions the clinician can pose to the individual:

- What do you need to work on in order to reach your VOR?
- What are your priorities for treatment?
- What do you need to learn or to do differently?

Objectives

Once the goals have been established, it is time to begin working on the specific steps that are needed to move toward reaching them. Objectives are behaviorally written and measureable. They tend to be most effective when they are stepwise and sequential.

This step is typically where individuals identify their barriers to more effective function-ing and are taught specific skills or coping strategies that they can apply in treatment and generalize to their lives. The timeframes for objectives are typically what the client will do each day or on a weekly basis. Progression may be to initially identify a pattern of functioning, identify strengths and barriers, teach the individual skills or coping strategies, have them apply them in the treatment setting, and assign homework for generalization with a tracking and review process. Homework and objectives need to be reviewed and worked on in each session to promote accountability and consistency. Here are a few examples of questions the clinician can pose to the individual:

- What do you need to work on each day in order to reach your goals?
- What should be the first step toward your goal? What comes next?
- How will you monitor your attempts to apply what you have learned and track whether it was effective?

Vision of Recovery

1. Goal: _____

    a. Objective (step 1): _____

    b. Objective (step 2): _____

    c. Objective (step 3): _____

2. Goal: _____

    a. Objective (step 1): _____

    b. Objective (step 2): _____

    c. Objective (step 3): _____

3. Goal: _____

    a. Objective (step 1): _____

    b. Objective (step 2): _____

    c. Objective (step 3): _____

NAME: _____

Goal Setting Homework

Step 1 – Define:

My *goal* is to: _____

My *need* is to: _____

Step 2 – Assets (What are the available resources you can use to achieve your goal?):

_____

_____

Step 3 – Barriers (What might get in the way of your achieving your goal?):

Barriers to my goal: _____

_____

Skills I can use: _____

_____

Step 4 – Action Plan (What are your behaviors and what is the timeline for each?):

Behavior: _____   Timeline: _____

Behavior: _____   Timeline: _____

Behavior: _____   Timeline: _____

Step 5 – Report the outcome in session:

What was the outcome? _____

_____

_____

_____

Biological Curriculum

Diary Card

	Rx	ANG	DEP	ANX	Stress Level	**Safety**	Positive Events	Use of Support System	Energy Level	Sleep Quality	Assertiveness	Efforts of Problem Solving	Today's Meaning	OTHER (MY GOALS)
MON														
RATING 0–10													1. 2. 3.	
Helpful Interventions														
TUE														
RATING 0–10													1. 2. 3.	
Helpful Interventions														
WED														
RATING 0–10													1. 2. 3.	
Helpful Interventions														
THU														
RATING 0–10													1. 2. 3.	
Helpful Interventions														
FRI														
RATING 0–10													1. 2. 3.	
Helpful Interventions														
SAT														
RATING 0–10													1. 2. 3.	
Helpful Interventions														
SUN														
RATING 0–10													1. 2. 3.	
Helpful Interventions														

Name: _____　　Week of Dates: _____ through _____

Stages of Change

The graph is designed to create categories for the individual to focus on. When distress is present, it may be difficult to understand the relationships they have between their distress and their functioning. This can provide insight and additional information to address in sessions. This graph can also show the complexity of relationships between distress and functioning while guiding the individual toward skill use.

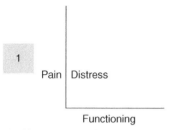

The X-axis is low to high levels of pain and the Y-axis is low to high functioning levels. When pain is present it causes distress, which in turn reduces functioning levels.

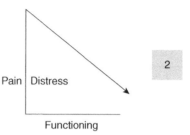

The goal is to decrease pain and increase functioning by reducing distress levels. The arrow indicates the goal of reducing pain and increasing functioning.

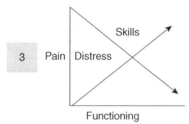

The mechanism of change is through the addition of skill use, which is represented by the arrow pointing upward. This indicates that functioning will increase when the individual becomes more effective with their skill use.

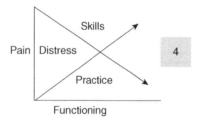

The key concept of practice is introduced to indicate that it takes time to practice new and existing skills to become more effective. Through consistent practice of the skills, distress will be reduced and functioning will be increased.

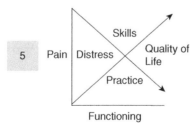

Quality of Life is now introduced. The more effective the individual's skill use becomes through practice, they will function at a higher level with less distress. The ending result is improved quality of life.

NAME: _____

Control versus Influence Homework

Control may be defined as having power over something (changing reality).

List 10 things you have control over.

1. _____
2. _____
3. _____
4. _____
5. _____
6. _____
7. _____
8. _____
9. _____
10. _____

Which aspects of your physical pain can you control?

_____

_____

Which aspects of your psychological distress can you control?

_____

_____

How do your physical pain and psychological distress affect each other?

_____

_____

Which aspects of the combination of physical pain and psychological distress do you have control over?

_____

_____

Influence may be defined as producing some effect without exerting direct control or power (making things better or worse).

List 10 things you can influence.

1. _____

2. _____

3. _____

4. _____

5. _____

6. _____

7. _____

8. _____

9. _____

10. _____

Which aspects of your physical pain can you influence?

_____

_____

Which aspects of your psychological distress can you influence?

_____

_____

How do your physical pain and psychological distress affect each other?

_____

_____

Which aspects of the combination of physical pain and psychological distress do you have influence over?

_____

_____

NAME: _____

Preparing for an Appointment Homework

1. Prioritize needs and wants – Brainstorm a sheet of needs and wants. Organize them into a list, with priorities at the top.

#1 NEED: _____ #1 WANT: _____

#2 NEED: _____ #2 WANT: _____

#3 NEED: _____ #3 WANT: _____

2. Set clear goals and objectives for the appointment – Know the purpose of the meeting and, specifically, what you want to accomplish before the meeting ends.

GOAL: _____

What I want to accomplish today: _____

3. Create a list of questions for the professional – Organize your thoughts into a list of questions. Post them in an area that you frequently spend time in so you can add questions to the list as you think of them.

Questions: _____ Answered? Y/N

_____ Answered? Y/N

_____ Answered? Y/N

4. Organize the tracking forms and tracking cards – Gather the most recent and relevant information you have. This is one way to avoid being forgetful or vague.

Do I have my Tracking Cards Ready? Y/N

Do I have all of the most recent information ready? Y/N

5. Plan for childcare, if needed – Ask a friend, family member, or the professional's facility to assist. It is important to be able to focus your attention and be mindful during the appointment.

Do I need someone to take care of my children? Y/N

If yes, who can I count on? _____

6. Plan or coordinate transportation – Make sure you have a reliable plan and mode of transportation. This is one of the main reasons individuals miss appointments.

Do I need transportation for this appointment? Y/N

If yes, who can I call? _____

7. Plan for an advocate to attend, if needed – You may want to ask a friend or family member to take notes during the appointment.

Do I need someone there at the appointment with me? Y/N

If yes, who can I count on? _____

8. Visualize the appointment – Imagine yourself staying focused, active, and productive in the meeting. This will help increase your chances of meeting your needs.

What will this appointment be like?

_____

_____

NAME: _____

Self-Advocacy Homework

Most of pain management is what you are willing to do, rather than what your doctors can do for you. Remember: it is your pain, not your doctor's pain. You must be an individual and an active participant in your life, not just a "patient."

1. What must be done in order for you to believe that all medical interventions or treatments have been tried?

_____

_____

_____

_____

2. What do you feel could be done now to improve your medical interventions or treatments?

_____

_____

_____

_____

3. Do you have all of the medical information necessary to make your decisions?

_____

_____

_____

_____

4. What information might you need, and where can you get it?

_____

_____

_____

_____

5. What are your thoughts or beliefs about your current medications?

_____

_____

_____

_____

6. Are your current medications effective?

_____

_____

_____

_____

7. Are you experiencing side effects that your doctors are aware of?

_____

_____

_____

_____

8. Do you believe that your medical team listens to you?

_____

_____

_____

_____

9. Does your medical team explain things so you can understand them?

_____

_____

_____

_____

10. What are your current priorities that your medical providers need to be aware of, and are they aware of them?

_____

_____

_____

_____

Baseline Assessment

1. **Establish a baseline of current pain through self-assessment** – This is where the individual rates their pain on a 10-point scale, with 10 being extreme pain and 0 being no pain. The individual then selects a level of pain that is acceptable to them and at which they have effective coping strategies.

2. **Review similar past activities by examining the frequency of engagement and how that affected pain levels** – This is where the individual recalls similar situations and compares their current functioning to previous functioning when engaging in similar activities. The comparison between past and present may provide information on how frequently they engage in activities before their pain levels are pushed to coping threshold. *If the probability of increased pain is high, the individual may need to decrease the frequency with which they engage in the activity.*

3. **Review similar past activities by examining the intensity of engagement and how that affected pain levels** – This is where the individual recalls similar situations and compares their current functioning to previous functioning when engaging in similar activities. The comparison between past and present may provide information on how intensely they engage in activities before their pain levels are pushed to coping threshold. *If the probability of increased pain is high, the individual may need to modify the intensity of the activity by pacing their engagement in it or by altering the activity itself.*

4. **Review similar past activities by examining the duration of engagement and how that affected pain levels** – This is where the individual recalls similar situations and compares their current functioning to previous functioning when engaging in similar activities. The comparison between past and present may provide information on how long they can engage in activities before their pain levels are pushed to coping threshold. *If the probability of increased pain is high, the individual may need to decrease the length of engagement in the activity. They may need to break the task into smaller parts that can be accomplished in stages over time.*

5. **Analyze the data and attempt to predict the pain response given past experience and current functioning and ability** – This is where the individual compares the present situation to what they have learned from the past. They create a probability for increased pain that is low, moderate, or high.

6. **Complete a pros and cons list for engagement in the activity versus non-engagement** – This is where the individual decides whether the "risk is worth the reward." They also review their current strengths and vulnerabilities.

7. **Create/review a skills implementation plan or coping plan** – This is where the individual creates or reviews a specific coping plan in relation to the activity.

8. **Create an action plan and commit to its implementation** – This is where the individual acts on their plan with no regret or remorse. They have done their best to analyze the situation and act accordingly.

NAME: _____

Baseline Assessment Homework

1. Establish a baseline of current pain through self-assessment

_____

_____

2. Review similar past activities by examining the frequency of engagement and how that affected pain levels

_____

_____

3. Review similar past activities by examining the intensity of engagement and how that affected pain levels

_____

_____

4. Review similar past activities by examining the duration of engagement and how that affected pain levels

_____

_____

5. Analyze the data and attempt to predict the pain response given past experience and current functioning and ability

_____

_____

6. Complete a pros and cons list for engagement in the activity versus non-engagement

	+	−
Engaging		
NOT Engaging	+	−

7. Create/review a skills implementation plan or coping plan

_____

_____

8. Create an action plan and commit to its implementation

_____

_____

Location of Pain

Date: _____

Time of Day (circle)	Activity (describe)	Intervention Used (check)	Level of Pain BEFORE Intervention (check)	Level of Pain AFTER Intervention (check)	Location of Pain (circle)

Morning:

12:00am–2:00am _____
2:00am–4:00am _____
4:00am–6:00am _____
6:00am–8:00am _____
8:00am–10:00am _____

Intervention Used (check):
☐ Used medication for pain (Biological)
☐ Used skills to manage pain (Psychological)
☐ Used support for pain (Social)
☐ No interventions

Level of Pain BEFORE Intervention (check):
10 9 8 7 6 5 4 3 2 1
☐ High (excruciating, difficulty functioning)
☐ Mild (some difficulty functioning)
☐ Low (noticeable, bothersome)

Level of Pain AFTER Intervention (check):
10 9 8 7 6 5 4 3 2 1
☐ High (excruciating, difficulty functioning)
☐ Mild (some difficulty functioning)
☐ Low (noticeable, bothersome)

Middary/Evening:

10:00am–12:00pm _____
12:00pm–2:00pm _____
2:00pm–4:00pm _____
4:00pm–6:00pm _____

Intervention Used (check):
☐ Used medication for pain (Biological)
☐ Used skills to manage pain (Psychological)
☐ Used support for pain (Social)
☐ No interventions

Level of Pain BEFORE Intervention (check):
10 9 8 7 6 5 4 3 2 1
☐ High (excruciating, difficulty functioning)
☐ Mild (some difficulty functioning)
☐ Low (noticeable, bothersome)

Level of Pain AFTER Intervention (check):
10 9 8 7 6 5 4 3 2 1
☐ High (excruciating, difficulty functioning)
☐ Mild (some difficulty functioning)
☐ Low (noticeable, bothersome)

Evening/Night:

6:00pm–8:00pm _____
8:00pm–10:00pm _____
10:00pm–12:00am _____

Intervention Used (check):
☐ Used medication for pain (Biological)
☐ Used skills to manage pain (Psychological)
☐ Used support for pain (Social)
☐ No interventions

Level of Pain BEFORE Intervention (check):
10 9 8 7 6 5 4 3 2 1
☐ High (excruciating, difficulty functioning)
☐ Mild (some difficulty functioning)
☐ Low (noticeable, bothersome)

Level of Pain AFTER Intervention (check):
10 9 8 7 6 5 4 3 2 1
☐ High (excruciating, difficulty functioning)
☐ Mild (some difficulty functioning)
☐ Low (noticeable, bothersome)

Location of Pain (circle)

NAME: _____

Behavior Chain Analysis Homework

What was the event? *(Who? What? When? Where?)*

_____

_____

_____

_____

What led up to the event? *(Give specifics of events, people, feelings, and beliefs)*

_____

_____

_____

_____

What did you gain or expect to gain by making your choice? *(Emotional, financial, relationships)*

_____

_____

_____

_____

What were the benefits you gained by making your choice?

_____

_____

_____

_____

What were the negative consequences of your choice? *(For yourself, for others)*

_____

_____

_____

_____

What skills could you use to intervene next time? *(What might you do/think differently?)*

_____

_____

_____

_____

Building a Healthy Sleep Routine

There are several elements to building a healthy sleep routine. The individual is encouraged to practice these elements for at least 1 month in a consistent manner.

1. **Go to bed when you are sleepy**
   Do not force your sleep. It may be helpful to set a consistent time to start your bedtime ritual that assists in preparing you for sleep.
2. **If you do not fall asleep after 20 minutes, you need to get out of bed**
   Find a distraction that does not involve strenuous activity and is short in duration. When you become sleepy, go back to bed. This may require a commitment to this process over and over until positive gains are achieved.
3. **Get out of bed at the same time every morning**
   You really want to minimize exceptions to this concept. Consistency is a stepping stone to healthy habits. The more we make exceptions, the harder and longer we have to work.
4. **Establish a bedtime ritual that helps you prepare for sleep**
   Engage in activities that calm the mind and body. Warm baths, scents, meditation, stretching, and reading are all effective examples. Notice that watching television is not on this list!
5. **Keep your bedroom cool, quiet, and dark**
   This promotes the 3 C's of sleep: cool, calm, and centered.
6. **Keep to your schedule**
   Creating healthy habits takes time and consistency. Over time, you will typically experience deeper, restorative sleep.
7. **Avoid naps if at all possible**
   If you must nap, keep it to 10–15 minutes in length.

Maintaining a Healthy Sleep Routine

1. **Bed is for sleep, so minimize other activities done in your bed**
   Your bed is for sleep, not talking on the phone, watching TV, eating, or working on the computer.
2. **Minimize or stop caffeine intake after mid-afternoon**
   This will assist in keeping you calm and relaxed.
3. **Avoid any alcohol consumption within 6 hours of bedtime**
   Alcohol and deep, restorative sleep do not mix well
4. **Avoid big meals or being too hungry before bedtime**
   It is important to have balance with hunger around bedtime. If you need to eat, moderation is key.
5. **Avoid exercising 6 hours before bedtime**
   Daily exercise is very important but needs to be done earlier in the day.
6. **Have a plan to cope with worry thoughts**
   Engage in deep breathing, visualization, or progressive muscle relaxation when agitated. Keep a notepad next to your bed to write your worry thoughts down and address them in the morning (practice letting go).
7. **List strategies to get back to sleep**
   Focus on relaxing your body and calming your mind. Engage in a quiet, nonstimulating activity.
8. **Consult your doctor**
   This is important to do before starting an exercise program, in order to assess whether your sleep problems require a primary medical intervention.

NAME: _____

Sleep Hygiene Homework

What steps do you need to take to improve your restorative sleep?

1. Preparation

_____

_____

_____

_____

2. If trouble occurs

_____

_____

_____

_____

3. When to wake up

_____

_____

_____

_____

4. Naps

_____

_____

_____

_____

5. Maintenance

_____

_____

_____

_____

Psychological Curriculum

Experiential Mapping

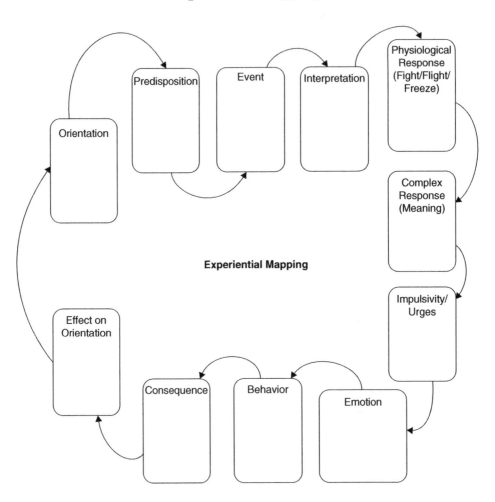

NAME: _____

Scheduling Positive Events Homework

	MORNING	AFTERNOON	EVENING	NIGHT
SELF				
OTHERS				

Guided Imagery

The Guided Imagery technique is a relaxation technique that allows you to refocus your attention away from your pain and symptoms and to promote calming, relaxing sensations. These sensations can be very helpful in reducing the intensity of pain, and they have the added benefit of inducing deep breathing and calming your body to a more relaxed state.

There are several ways in which to use the Guided Imagery technique. You could picture a place and imagine the details by yourself. Or, you could have a friend or family member read Guided Imagery scripts. Alternatively, you could listen to a recording of a script. Each method provides a different experience, promoting feelings of calmness and relaxation. You can learn new places to visualize, or even create your own images, allowing a personalized experience of relaxation.

Scene for Guided Imagery

Take this time now to allow yourself to quiet your mind and focus on something other than the current moment. Allow yourself to be seated comfortably and begin to focus on your breaths. Notice the breaths you take as you begin to relax comfortably.

Begin to build an image in your mind now of a place where you are fully relaxed. This place is yours to experience, and no one can bother you in this place. Imagine yourself standing in the grass on a steep hill. The grass is cool, prickly, and wet on your bare feet. As you stand at the top of this steep hill, you feel the warmth of the sun soaking through your shirt on to your back, toasting the skin on your neck. As you look down the hill, you notice a small object, unclear of what it is.

As you proceed down the hill, you walk slowly, feeling the prickle of the cool, wet grass beneath your feet. You begin by taking small steps, increasing your strides with the steep hill, feeling the pressure on your thighs and knees as you proceed slowly down the hill.

Once you approach the object, you notice it is a small, purple flower with yellow pollen. The flower has four small, almond-shaped pedals. As you kneel down to be closer to the flower, you feel a cool, crisp breeze that blows your hair over your forehead. As you reach up to swipe the hair away, you notice the warmth of your fingertips touching your skin. As you look up, you notice more purple flowers, leading around a group of tall trees. As you begin to follow the path of the flowers, you notice a shadow behind the trees.

As you approach the end of the group of trees, you feel the coolness of the shade the trees provide. With the sun now absent from view, you notice the hairs on your arm standing up in response to the coolness of the shade. Looking down, you begin to smell the scent of the purple flowers: a light, sweet scent of flora. You begin to follow the trickling trail of purple flowers and notice once again the shaded object ahead.

As you approach the object, you see that is a brick wall – a rounded, tall, brick wall. As you walk closer to the brick wall, you place your hand up against it, feeling the bumps, ridges, and cracks in the rough brick. As you pick up speed, you can see the brick wall comes to an end. At the end of the brick wall, you can see a tall iron gate. Once you reach the gate, your hands grasp around the cool, hard iron, and you feel the metal against your fingertips. Using your hands, you push the gate open, hearing the creaking squeal of the gate opening.

As you proceed through the gate, you notice a sound: a distant bubbling sound of water. As you follow the sound, you begin to smell the water: the cool, musty smell of fresh water. As you grow closer and closer to the water, you finally set eyes on a small, babbling creek. As you walk closer and closer to the creek, you hear the noises of the bubbling water. Approaching the creek, you bend down to take a drink, feeling the pressure of the rocks on your knees. Dipping your hand into the creek, you feel the sharp, cold water against your hand and sweep the water up to your mouth. Taking a drink, you feel the cold water traveling down your throat, quenching your thirst.

Now that you are refreshed, you begin back toward the iron gate, walking past the tall brick wall, through the trail of purple flowers, and back up the hill, feeling your muscles worked, your thirst quenched, and your mind relaxed.

Take another deep breath and return to the moment, when you are ready.

Tips for Guided Imagery

- If at any point you become uncomfortable, distracted, or discouraged, stop Guided Imagery.
- Start at a time where you can dedicate a few moments to relaxation.
- Remember to breathe – count on your body's natural rhythm to keep you steady.
- Try various scenes in order to promote sensations from each of your five senses.

(Adapted from Hamann, 2015)

Progressive Muscle Relaxation

This is one of the most widely used techniques that can assist in controlling symptoms. The process of tensing and relaxing muscles is easy and can be individualized to fit specific needs. One of the reasons muscle relaxation is so effective is that it produces immediate physical results, which help you recognize tension and release it, leading to better control of bodily pain. Another reason is that it is easy to learn and easy to practice across different settings. For example, it can be used at work or at home, and sitting or standing. Among its effects are increased relaxation, reduced muscle tension, increased calmness, and reduced overall pain.

There are many ways to practice muscle relaxation.

Start by sitting or standing in a comfortable position. Give yourself time to focus upon your own body. The point of this exercise is to locate, identify, and experience tension and relaxation. Try to let all other noises and distractions go by closing your eyes – this is *your* time to focus on *your* body.

Technique for Progressive Muscle Relaxation

First, begin by taking several deep breaths, comfortably filling your lungs with air and noticing your chest rise as it fills with air. Begin to notice your abdomen as it fills with air. First your chest rises, and then your abdomen raises as you fill your body with air. Notice your breath, breathing slowly in…and out again. Take a moment to notice your breath.

Now begin to focus your attention on your lower body. Notice your feet, the feet that carry your body. Notice the feeling in your feet. Begin to tense your feet now, curling your toes under, squeezing each muscle in your feet. HOLD this tension…

Now relax your feet. Notice the feeling between tension and relaxation. Next, notice the muscles in your lower legs, your calves, your shins, and your knees. Begin to tense your lower legs by tightening the muscles in your calves, shins, and knees. HOLD this tension…

Now relax your lower legs. Notice the feeling between tension and relaxation. Next, notice the muscles in your upper legs, your hamstrings and buttocks. Begin to tense your upper legs by tightening your hamstrings, thighs, and buttocks and squeeze these muscles. HOLD this tension…

Now relax your upper legs. Notice the difference between tension and relaxation in both of your legs, from your thighs to your feet. Now notice your abdomen, the place in your body that houses your organs, which give your life. Begin to tense your abdomen by squeezing your stomach muscles, your obliques, your sides and back, pulling yourself upward and tightening the core of your body. HOLD this tension…

Now release and relax. Notice the feeling between tension and relaxation, the difference between tension and relaxation. Now notice the muscles in your arms, your wrists, triceps, and biceps. Begin to tense these muscles by squeezing only your arms and tightening the muscles in your arms. HOLD this tension…

Now relax your arms, noticing the difference between tension and relaxation. Now notice your hands. Your hands, which are so useful to you. Begin to squeeze your hands together by making tight fists, using each finger, palm, and thumb of your hands, tightening them together. HOLD this tension…

Relax your hands, noticing the difference between tension and relaxation. Now, focus your attention on your neck. Your neck, which holds your head. Begin by tightening the muscles in your neck and squeezing those muscles. Squeeze your shoulder blades together and notice the tension. HOLD this tension…

Now relax your neck. Notice the feeling between tension and relaxation. Lastly, focus your attention on your face. Begin to tighten the muscles in your face, your cheeks, around your eyes, mouth, and forehead, and tighten your face. HOLD this tension…

And now relax your face. Notice now the amount of energy your body uses to create the feeling of tension. Focus on the difference between the feeling of tension and the feeling of relaxation. Notice now your body completely relaxed. Your feet, legs, abdomen, arms, neck, and face, all relaxed. Allow yourself to enjoy the feeling of relaxation…Take another deep breath now, allowing your chest to rise with air, and slowly open your eyes and return back to the moment.

Tips for Progressive Muscle Relaxation

- If pain becomes intense, reduce the amount of tension you create.
- Let go of distractions, even if you hear noises or remember tasks uncompleted. Allow yourself these few moments to relax and focus on your own body.
- Once you feel comfortable with relaxing your entire body, focus on the area of pain in order to relieve the pain effectively.
- Pick a quiet place and a quiet time.
- Set realistic expectations for yourself and your relaxation.
- Remember to practice.

(Adapted from Hamann, 2015)

NAME:_____

Meditation

Type	Steps for Meditation or Relaxation
Guided meditation	With the help of a teacher or guide, or even a pre-made recording, take yourself on a journey through a place you find calming or relaxing. Visualize your surroundings, and try to incorporate as many senses as possible. Soak in the sounds, smells, and textures.
Mantra, or transcendental meditation	Choose a calming word or phrase. Repeat it silently over and over to yourself to prevent distracting thoughts from entering.
Mindful meditation	Take a break and make yourself acutely aware of your surroundings. Take deep breaths and feel your lungs swell. Allow yourself to think about your feelings, but do so without judgment.
Yoga or tai chi	Perform a slow series of varying postures while breathing deeply. As you balance and move, focus on the movements and not on the stress in your life. Attend a class to learn the basics. Then you can practice in your own home.
Prayer	Pray using your own words, or read prayers written by others. Reflect on the meaning of the words or write in a journal.
Deep breathing	Take deep breaths from your diaphragm, rather than short, shallow breaths from your chest. Continue until you feel calm.
Biofeedback	This involves a doctor attaching electrodes to your body in order to monitor blood pressure, breathing, heart rate, and muscle tension. A therapist will then study your reactions and teach you how to reduce the types of stress you experience.
Exercise	Try going for a walk or run to clear your mind and reduce stress.

(Adapted from www.wikihow.com)

Coping with Stress

- **Acting out** – Coping with stress by engaging in actions rather than reflections or feelings.
  - o Healthy – Feeling high levels of distress and turning energy toward walking, working out, or completing tasks.
  - o Unhealthy – Throwing temper tantrums, acting impulsively, being aggressive.
- **Affiliation** – Turning to other people for support.
  - o Healthy – Sharing experience with others, asking for support or validation.
  - o Unhealthy – Having others do things one could do oneself, becoming dependent on others, losing independence.
- **Altruism** – Meeting internal needs through helping others.
  - o Healthy – Feeling high levels of distress and distracting oneself by helping a friend or neighbor, volunteering time, becoming active in the community or an organization.
  - o Unhealthy – Putting others' needs before one's own or engaging in self-neglect.
- **Avoidance** – Refusing to deal with or encounter unpleasant situations or objects.
  - o Healthy – Feeling high levels of distress and taking a break, distracting oneself for brief periods, doing something nice for oneself.
  - o Unhealthy – Sticking one's head in the sand, pretending things don't exist, escaping/avoiding/altering the distress.
- **Compensation** – Overachieving in one area to compensate for failures in another.
  - o Healthy – Feeling high levels of distress and turning energy toward things one does well, applying the **Building Mastery** skill, doing things to feel competent.
  - o Unhealthy – Masking, engaging in things one does well to falsely appear competent, pretending one is doing well when one is not.
- **Denial** – Refusing to acknowledge or recognize reality (individuals who abuse drugs or alcohol often deny that they have a problem, while victims of traumatic events may deny that the event ever occurred).
  - o Healthy – Feeling high levels of distress and applying the skill Push Away (**ACCEPTS**), leaving a situation for a short period of time with a plan to return and address the distress later.
  - o Unhealthy – Leaving a situation with no plan to return or to address the distress, denying what is real and letting problems build, invalidating one's own experience.
- **Devaluation** – Dealing with distress by attributing exaggerated negative qualities to oneself or others.
  - o Healthy – Feeling high levels of distress and applying the skill Comparisons (see **ACCEPTS**) to aspects or objects of the situation in order to take small steps toward addressing the situation or distress.
  - o Unhealthy – Decreasing one's self-esteem, hurting others, or minimizing the impact of the distress.
- **Displacement** – Taking out frustrations, feelings, and impulses on people or objects that are less powerful or less threatening.

- o Healthy – Feeling high levels of distress and punching a pillow, tearing a phone book, holding an ice cube.
- o Unhealthy – Destroying property, "kicking the dog," making others feel miserable.
- **Projection** – Falsely attributing unacceptable feelings, impulses, or thoughts to others.
  - o Healthy – Identifying with feelings of being cool, calm, and calculating in others, treating others with respect even when they are not being respectful back.
  - o Unhealthy – Denying one's own experience by placing it on others, fearing someone will leave and blaming them for being distant, feeling frustrated and accusing others of being angry.
- **Rationalization** – Explaining an unacceptable behavior or feeling in a rational or logical manner, while avoiding the true reasons for engaging in it.
  - o Healthy – Feeling high levels of distress and focusing on what one is doing well, engaging in positive self-talk, riding the wave of the current emotion, or reminding oneself that the distress will not last forever.
  - o Unhealthy – Blaming others, attributing failure to the personal qualities of others, devaluing others when one feels hurt or rejected, or labeling one's behavior as acceptable because others would act the same way.
- **Regression** – Abandoning coping strategies and returning to patterns of behavior used earlier in development.
  - o Healthy – Simplifying one's life for a short period of time, self-soothing, asking others for support and validation, or having others take care of one's needs for a short period in order to take a break from distress.
  - o Unhealthy – Throwing temper tantrums, locking oneself in one's room, becoming impulsive, or acting out.

(Adapted from American Psychiatric Association, 2013)

NAME:_____

Beliefs about Anger Homework

Validate each statement, finding an aspect that is true for you. Challenge each statement by finding when it is untrue for you, or provide a skill to use in order to increase your effective coping strategies.

1. My anger controls me.

    a. Validation statement _____

    b. Challenge statement _____

2. I deserve better than this.

    a. Validation statement _____

    b. Challenge statement _____

3. I go from calm to angry in seconds.

    a. Validation statement _____

    b. Challenge statement _____

4. Anger is the same as aggression.

    a. Validation statement _____

    b. Challenge statement _____

5. I shouldn't be so angry.

    a. Validation statement _____

    b. Challenge statement _____

6. My anger scares me.

    a. Validation statement _____

    b. Challenge statement _____

7. My anger can't be predicted.

    a. Validation statement _____

    b. Challenge statement _____

8. My anger can't be controlled.

    a. Validation statement _____

    b. Challenge statement _____

9. My anger protects me.

   a. Validation statement _____

   b. Challenge statement _____

10. Nothing helps to calm me down.

    a. Validation statement _____

    b. Challenge statement _____

11. Other…

    a. Validation statement _____

    b. Challenge statement _____

NAME:_____

Managing Conflict Homework

The skill set of **MAD** (M) is designed to manage conflict as it occurs. This skill set is similar to taking a timeout and interrupts the process of intense conflict.

- **M**inimize – Acknowledge that conflict is occurring and minimize the chances of acting from a state of anger. Go to a different room or location, let the other person know when you will return to continue working on the issue, and find ways to "cool off."
- **A**ssess – Identify the level of your emotional distress and the intensity of the engagement. Prioritize the skills of DM, G, and F. Create a plan to re-engage when you and the other person are *both* ready to continue. If the situation is still intense, repeat the first skill until a safe and productive conversation can occur.
- **D**amage control – Do not engage in hurtful words or actions. Do not allow yourself to be hurt or treated in a disrespectful manner. Repeat the two previous skills as needed.

1. What skills can you use to prepare for interactions that might lead to conflict?

_____

_____

_____

_____

2. How will you know when to use your **MAD** skills?

_____

_____

_____

_____

3. How will you know if your skills are effective?

_____

_____

_____

_____

4. Prepare your plan for potential conflict.

_____

_____

_____

_____

Taking a Timeout

Conflict and anger are natural parts of life that happen in all relationships. When anger presents as a barrier to effective communication, taking a timeout can interrupt an unhealthy or unproductive interaction.

1. Before the interaction, assess your emotional state.
    o   What are your feelings and how intensely are you feeling them?
2. Recognize when your emotions are intensifying from frustration toward anger. Catching yourself early in the process provides choice.
    o   Are your emotions matching what is needed in the current situation? Is the situation becoming too intense?
3. If you notice that your anger is increasing, remove yourself from the situation as soon as you can.
    o   Is now the time to take a timeout? Can you take a timeout safely?
4. If the situation involves another person, tell them that you need a timeout. Be cautious not to just leave. Use assertive "I" statements. Avoid blaming the other person and advocate for yourself. "I need some space" or "I need a break" is much more productive than assigning blame. Tell the other person when you plan on returning and explain why you currently need to disengage: "I need 10 minutes and a quiet space to calm down so I don't say anything I might regret."
    o   How do you separate yourself respectfully and in a calm manner?
5. Take a break and get some space from the situation.
    o   What do you need in order to follow through with your plan?
6. Once you have identified your needs and the actions you are going to take, engage in calming exercises. It is time to cool down.
    o   What do you need to do in order to calm your mind, body, and emotions?
7. While on your break, plan what you would like to say. It is important to act through the three C's: be Cool, be Clear, and be Concise.
    o   When you re-engage, what do you want to do or say, and how do you want to do or say it?
8. Once your anger and tension have reduced to a more manageable level, it is time to re-engage in the process. Keep in mind that you may be more prone to escalation, since this has already occurred at least once. You may need to repeat some of the previous steps.
    o   Are you ready, and do you have a realistic plan for success?
9. Re-engage by thanking the other person for being a part of a healthier process and follow your plan.
    o   Are you maintaining your effectiveness?

NAME:_____

Defense Mechanisms and Coping Styles Homework

Provide an example of how you relate to each of the following coping styles. To each unhealthy style, attach one skill that you can use to improve your attempts to cope more effectively. Remember: these are common to most individuals. Challenge any judgment you may have.

- **Acting out** – Coping with stress by engaging in actions rather than reflections or feelings.

    o Healthy _____

    o Unhealthy _____

- **Affiliation** – Turning to other people for support.

    o Healthy _____

    o Unhealthy _____

- **Altruism** – Meeting internal needs through helping others.

    o Healthy _____

    o Unhealthy _____

- **Avoidance** – Refusing to deal with or encounter unpleasant situations or objects.

    o Healthy _____

    o Unhealthy _____

- **Compensation** – Overachieving in one area to compensate for failures in another.

    o Healthy _____

    o Unhealthy _____

- **Denial** – Refusing to acknowledge or recognize reality (individuals who abuse drugs or alcohol often deny that they have a problem, while victims of traumatic events may deny that the event ever occurred).

    o Healthy _____

    o Unhealthy _____

- **Devaluation** – Dealing with distress by attributing exaggerated negative qualities to oneself or others.

  - Healthy _____

  - Unhealthy _____

- **Displacement** – Taking out frustrations, feelings, and impulses on people or objects that are less powerful or less threatening.

  - Healthy _____

  - Unhealthy _____

- **Projection** – Falsely attributing unacceptable feelings, impulses, or thoughts to others.

  - Healthy _____

  - Unhealthy _____

- **Rationalization** – Explaining an unacceptable behavior or feeling in a rational or logical manner, while avoiding the true reasons for engaging in it.

  - Healthy _____

  - Unhealthy _____

- **Regression** – Abandoning coping strategies and returning to patterns of behavior used earlier in development.

  - Healthy _____

  - Unhealthy _____

NAME:_____

Finding Meaning and Purpose Homework
Physical Pain

Individuals relate first to their physical environment, which includes their body. When pain is present, it affects functioning. They may experience limitations, changes in abilities, financial problems, and increased risk of injury or illness.

Lack of meaning and purpose: _____

_____

_____

_____

_____

Meaning and purpose: _____

_____

_____

_____

_____

Social Pain

Humans are social beings. Individuals relate to others in their world. This category includes relationships, cultural issues, socioeconomic issues, race identity, conflict with others, competition issues, and failure.

Lack of meaning and purpose: _____

_____

_____

_____

_____

Meaning and purpose: _____

_____

_____

_____

_____

Psychological Pain

The psychological category includes how individuals relate to themselves and their own personal sense of identity.

Lack of meaning and purpose: _____

_____

_____

_____

_____

Meaning and purpose: _____

_____

_____

_____

_____

Spiritual Pain

This category includes the individual's attitude toward the unknown and how they assign meaning to experiences. This category also includes the individual's sense of connection, which is up to each individual to define.

Lack of meaning and purpose: _____

_____

_____

_____

_____

Meaning and purpose: _____

_____

_____

_____

_____

NAME:_____

First Steps toward Change Homework

- **Just Noticeable Change** (JNC) – Engaging in a behavior that leads to a change in focus or direction.

This is a "baby-steps" skill, providing a first step toward change. It is designed to change the individual's "threshold" of experience. This helps them identify that small steps can have a big impact on the process of change.

Provide an example that you want to maintain or reinforce in each of the following categories.

Thoughts: _____

_____

_____

_____

_____

Feelings: _____

_____

_____

_____

_____

Behaviors: _____

_____

_____

_____

_____

Attitudes: _____

_____

_____

_____

_____

Expectations: _____

_____

_____

_____

_____

Beliefs: _____

_____

_____

_____

_____

Anticipated outcomes: _____

_____

_____

_____

_____

Provide an example that you want to take the first step toward changing in each of the following categories. Include your first step.

Thoughts: _____

_____

_____

_____

_____

Feelings: _____

_____

_____

_____

_____

Behaviors: _____

_____

_____

_____

_____

Attitudes: _____

_____

_____

_____

_____

Expectations: _____

_____

_____

_____

_____

Beliefs: _____

_____

_____

_____

_____

Anticipated outcomes: _____

_____

_____

_____

_____

NAME:_____

Challenging Stigma Homework

1. Pain is a way to escape reality (avoidance)

    o Validation statement _____

    o Challenge statement _____

2. You are not tough enough (weakness)

    o Validation statement _____

    o Challenge statement _____

3. You are not motivated enough (resistant)

    o Validation statement _____

    o Challenge statement _____

4. You don't want to be fixed (broken)

    o Validation statement _____

    o Challenge statement _____

5. You should…(invalidating)

    o Validation statement _____

    o Challenge statement _____

6. You are living off the government (freeloader)

    o Validation statement _____

    o Challenge statement _____

7. You're making yourself hurt so you can get drugs (addict)

    o Validation statement _____

    o Challenge statement _____

8. You are just a whiner (weakness)

    o Validation statement _____

    o Challenge statement _____

9. You are trying to avoid work (lazy)

    o Validation statement _____

    o Challenge statement _____

10. You are trying to get attention (needy)

    o Validation statement _____

    o Challenge statement _____

11. Your pain is not real – it's all in your head (faking)

    o Validation statement _____

    o Challenge statement _____

12. You're not really that bad off (catastrophizing)

    o Validation statement _____

    o Challenge statement _____

13. Your pain flares up at convenient times (manipulation)

    o Validation statement _____

    o Challenge statement _____

14. Other people are doing better than you are (minimizing)

    o Validation statement _____

    o Challenge statement _____

15. You are "crazy," "nuts," or a "psycho (devaluating)

    o Validation statement _____

    o Challenge statement _____

Social Curriculum

NAME:_____

Intimacy in Relationships Homework

How do you define intimacy in your relationships?

_____
_____
_____
_____

What actions do you take to promote intimacy?

_____
_____
_____
_____

What actions would you like to engage in more often?

_____
_____
_____
_____

How do you anticipate others reacting?

_____
_____
_____
_____

How will this affect your relationships?

_____
_____
_____
_____

What is your plan to promote intimacy?

_____

_____

_____

_____

How will you know if your plan is working? (Review problem-solving models)

_____

_____

_____

_____

Commit to your plan!

NAME:_____

Exploring Roles and Responsibilities Homework

For each of the following roles, provide a positive and a challenge of adapting that role.

- **Blamer** – For the blamer, when things go wrong, someone is to blame. Energy and focus may be spent on the negative consequences, and not necessarily on the individual's responsibility.
  - o Positives _____
  - o Challenges _____
- **Cheerleader** – The cheerleader encourages others with great enthusiasm. Individuals typically functioning within this role tend to be positive and popular with others.
  - o Positives _____
  - o Challenges _____
- **Distracter** – The distracter draws attention away from problems and toward things that are easier to accept and handle. Those around them may experience a release from responsibility or reality for a brief period of time.
  - o Positives _____
  - o Challenges _____
- **Favored son** – The favored son has a special place in the hearts of parental figures or those in authority. They are given positives continually, whether deserved or not.
  - o Positives _____
  - o Challenges _____
- **Hero** – The hero finds a way to save the day when things go wrong or people are threatened. They help both people in distress and those around them.
  - o Positives _____
  - o Challenges _____
- **Invalid** – The invalid is sick, injured, or otherwise limited in some capacity, sometimes through their own choice. They are often a burden on others, who feel obligated to help them.
  - o Positives _____
  - o Challenges _____
- **Jester** – The jester finds humor or levity in most situations. This role helps people avoid emotionally difficult situations.
  - o Positives _____
  - o Challenges _____

- **Martyr** – The martyr experiences pain and suffering with little complaint. They are willing to make sacrifices for their beliefs or those around them. A distinctive benefit is the receipt of sympathetic attention from others.
    - Positives _____
    - Challenges _____
- **Mascot** – The mascot is a good-luck symbol for a family. They are often loved and accepted by others for the positive feelings they give to those around them.
    - Positives _____
    - Challenges _____
- **Placator** – The placator dissipates conflict between others and can help others resolve their issues. It is common for them to focus on the problems of others in order to distract from their own difficulties.
    - Positives _____
    - Challenges _____
- **Rebel** – The rebel thinks and functions outside of accepted systems and processes. They are autonomous and free spirits.
    - Positives _____
    - Challenges _____
- **Saint** – The saint is the epitome of all things good. They are unwavering in their positive approaches to others and to life in general.
    - Positives _____
    - Challenges _____
- **Scapegoat** – The scapegoat takes blame for things they both have and have not done. They may feel like a martyr, but are not treated in that manner by others.
    - Positives _____
    - Challenges _____
- **Skeptic** – The skeptic doubts and questions everything and everyone around them. When they do this in a healthy manner, they may find hope when others do not. However, they may also deny the truth when it is present.
    - Positives _____
    - Challenges _____
- **Star** – The star is given special status and adoration. Limitations are often minimized and strengths are maximized.
    - Positives _____
    - Challenges _____

(Adapted from Blevins, 1993)

NAME:_____

Individual-Based Problem-Solving Homework

The first strategy is for the individual who is addressing a problem without the involvement of others. This is done in a series of steps, some of which may need to be repeated and modified throughout the process.

1. Identify the problem _____

   a. How is this impacting your thoughts, feelings, and behaviors?

   _____

   _____

   _____

   _____

2. Review your values _____

   a. Include your strengths and limitations.

   _____

   _____

   _____

   _____

   b. This includes yourself, others, and your environment (systems you are involved with).

   _____

   _____

   _____

   _____

3. Brainstorm potential solutions _____

   a. Don't throw out any possibility.

   _____

   _____

   _____

   _____

4. Consider the potential consequences of each decision _____

    a. Narrow the possibilities and attach potential positive and negative conse-
        quences to each idea.

        _____

        _____

        _____

        _____

    b. Create a pros and cons list for each potential solution.

        _____

        _____

        _____

        _____

5. Select and implement a desired course of action _____

    a. Evaluate whether the plan is working and needs to be continued, or is not
        working as planned and needs to be modified of stopped.

        _____

        _____

        _____

        _____

NAME:_____

Social-Based Problem-Solving Homework

The second strategy is for the individual who is addressing a problem with the involvement of others. This is done in a series of steps, some of which may need to be repeated and modified throughout the process.

1. Recognize the problem _____

   a. What is the problem?

      _____

      _____

      _____

   b. Why is it a problem?

      _____

      _____

      _____

   c. Who is involved, both now and potentially in the future?

      _____

      _____

      _____

2. Define the problem _____

   a. Create your own definition.

      _____

      _____

      _____

   b. Consider factors of age, race, gender, values, and power differentials.

      _____

      _____

      _____

    c.   Get information and perspectives from others.

_____

_____

_____

3. Generate potential solutions _____

    a.   Brainstorm potential solutions.

_____

_____

_____

    b.   Create a pros and cons list for each.

_____

_____

_____

4. Select a potential solution _____

    a.   Consider whether the solution meets short-, mid-, or long-term needs.

_____

_____

_____

_____

5. Review the process _____

    a.   How did you reach this solution?

_____

_____

_____

    b.   Is the "golden rule" involved?

_____

_____

_____

c. Did you consider all relevant factors?

_____

_____

_____

d. What is your motivation for your decision?

_____

_____

_____

6. Implement and evaluate the solution _____

a. Is new information available?

_____

_____

_____

b. Do you need to continue, modify, or stop the plan?

_____

_____

_____

7. Reflect on the process _____

a. What was learned?

_____

_____

_____

b. How does this affect others, your environment, and yourself in the future?

_____

_____

_____

NAME:_____

Nurturing Support Systems Homework

There are many barriers to nurturing support systems. This list identifies some common examples and the potential hidden messages attached to each.

- "I am too busy." (You are not worth the effort.)
    - Validation statement _____
    - Challenge statement _____
- "I never thought of it." (I don't consider your needs to be a priority – I am too focused on myself.)
    - Validation statement _____
    - Challenge statement _____
- "They don't want anything from me" or "I have nothing to offer." (I am not worthy of them.)
    - Validation statement _____
    - Challenge statement _____
- "We fight all the time." (It is easier to avoid the individual or the situation [passive-aggressive].)
    - Validation statement _____
    - Challenge statement _____
- "Our relationship never needed this before." (I want things to be like they were.)
    - Validation statement _____
    - Challenge statement _____
- "I am in too much pain or distress to do this now." (It's not worth the effort.)
    - Validation statement _____
    - Challenge statement _____
- "I can't." (I don't know how.)
    - Validation statement _____
    - Challenge statement _____

- "I can't." (I don't want to.)

  - Validation statement _____

  - Challenge statement _____

- "I won't." (I can do this by myself.)

  - Validation statement _____

  - Challenge statement _____

- "I don't know how." (It is easier to avoid than to learn.)

  - Validation statement _____

  - Challenge statement _____

- "When should I do it?" (It's not convenient for me.)

  - Validation statement _____

  - Challenge statement _____

- "I don't have money to spend on them." (I can only show caring by buying gifts.)

  - Validation statement _____

  - Challenge statement _____

- "I just want to be left alone." (Let me suffer in isolation [martyr].)

  - Validation statement _____

  - Challenge statement _____

- "Things are just fine the way that they are now." (Denying reality.)

  - Validation statement _____

  - Challenge statement _____

NAME:_____

Remoralization Homework

Remoralization may be defined as instilling a sense of competency, hope, and connect-edness in individuals. This is a process that takes time, effort, and energy. Just as you did not become demoralized overnight, so remoralization will also take time.

Thoughts

How do my thoughts get in the way of doing what needs to be done?

_____

_____

Am I engaging in catastrophizing or minimizing thoughts?

_____

_____

Is there an "I don't know" response? (Not knowing HOW to do something and not WANTING to do something).

_____

_____

Feelings

How do my feelings get in the way of doing what needs to be done?

_____

_____

Behaviors

How do my actions (behaviors) get in the way of doing what needs to be done?

_____

_____

Attitudes

How do my attitudes (how I mentally approach a situation or life in general) get in the way of doing what needs to be done?

_____

_____

Do I have:

- Optimism – Interpreting and approaching situations in a positive manner?
- Pessimism – Interpreting and approaching situations in a skeptical manner?
- Willingness – Being quick to act or respond?
- Willfulness – Being intentionally self-willed or stubborn?

Expectations

How do my expectations get in the way of doing what needs to be done? (Self and others.)

_____

_____

Beliefs

How do my beliefs get in the way of doing what needs to be done?

_____

_____

- Identify the belief (e.g. "I am not capable of change") _____

  _____

- Identify the extreme stance (e.g. Not being capable) _____

  _____

- Find the kernel of truth (e.g. Change is a natural part of life/Few things never change) _____

  _____

- Identify the challenge (e.g. Change is difficult) _____

  _____

- Restate the new belief (e.g. "Change is hard for me") _____

  _____

Anticipated outcomes

How does what I anticipate happening get in the way of doing what needs to be done?

_____

_____

Active Listening

1. **Pay attention** – Be aware of your body language. Make eye contact and focus your attention on the other individual.
    o *Example: Turn your body toward the person, look at their face, and notice your body while in the conversation.*
2. **Be non-judgmental** – Keep an open mind. Be open to new ideas and perspectives. Avoid criticizing and arguing.
    o *Example: Take in their information and really listen. Avoid your ideas about the situation unless asked. Take in their information as new and interesting, and think about it.*
3. **Use reflective communication** – Paraphrase key points that the other person is making. Reflect back to them what you have heard to promote understanding and interaction.
    o *Example: "So, what I hear you saying is that you feel _____ because _____. Is that right?"*
4. **Ask questions** – Avoid making assumptions. Get clarity and encourage the other person to expand on their ideas.
    o *Example: "Do you feel angry about that?" "What was that like for you?" "Do you mean that you felt disappointed?"*
5. **Summarize** – Briefly restate the main points of what you have understood the other person to say.
    o *Example: "You're saying you're upset about the situation." "You felt hurt by that."*
6. **Reciprocate** – Share your experiences and how you can relate to others. Keep it brief.
    o *Example: "I have felt hurt like that before. How are you coping with that?" "I have experienced something like that before and I felt worried. What is it like for you?"*

Styles of Interacting Homework

- **Personalizing** – An individual who overidentifies with the presented information and perceives that others are talking about them or that they are to blame for something.
  - Need being met _____
  - Potential social barrier _____
  - Alternative action strategy _____

- **Fixing** – An individual who typically provides solutions to other people's problems even when solutions have not been requested.
  - Need being met _____
  - Potential social barrier _____
  - Alternative action strategy _____

- **Cheerleading** – An individual who encourages others by being overly optimistic and attempts to provide motivation to others in an unwavering manner.
  - Need being met _____
  - Potential social barrier _____
  - Alternative action strategy _____

- **Invalidating** – An individual who fails to connect to another person's experience and challenges or argues about what they "should" be experiencing.
  - Need being met _____
  - Potential social barrier _____
  - Alternative action strategy _____

- **Joining** – An individual who connects with other people through their pain or distress.
  - Need being met _____
  - Potential social barrier _____
  - Alternative action strategy _____

- **Tangential** – An individual who responds to others by connecting to minimally relevant aspects of the process or content of the interaction.
  - Need being met _____
  - Potential social barrier _____
  - Alternative action strategy _____

- **Competition** – An individual who challenges others by competing with their stories and identifies as being better or worse than others in some aspect of their disclosures.
  - o Need being met _____
  - o Potential social barrier _____
  - o Alternative action strategy _____
- **Masking** – An individual who hides or disguises their true experience and typically provides information that is not accurate to their own experience.
  - o Need being met _____
  - o Potential social barrier _____
  - o Alternative action strategy _____
- **Performing** – An individual who agrees with all feedback and challenges on a superficial level, and then either rejects change or attributes positives/blame to others.
  - o Need being met _____
  - o Potential social barrier _____
  - o Alternative action strategy _____
- **Externalizing** – An individual who attributes credit for success or failure to others in a consistent manner.
  - o Need being met _____
  - o Potential social barrier _____
  - o Alternative action strategy _____
- **Help-rejecting complaining** – An individual who identifies a problem and then dismisses all potential solutions.
  - o Need being met _____
  - o Potential social barrier _____
  - o Alternative action strategy _____
- **Finding extremes** – An individual who uses extremes in language, thoughts, or behaviors.
  - o Need being met _____
  - o Potential social barrier _____
  - o Alternative action strategy _____
- **Emotional sponging** – An individual who adopts the emotions of those around them as their own.
  - o Need being met _____
  - o Potential social barrier _____
  - o Alternative action strategy _____

NAME:_____

The 3 I's Homework

Identity, Insecurity, Isolation

What is the issue you need to focus on? *(Identify and define the challenge)*

_____

_____

_____

_____

Why is this currently a challenge in your life? *(Want or need, for self or others, or both)*

_____

_____

_____

_____

What do you hope to gain by working on this challenge? *(Emotional, financial, relationships, stability)*

_____

_____

_____

_____

What are your current resources and what supports do you have? *(List your strengths and things/people that can help you)*

_____

_____

_____

_____

What are the current barriers to accessing your resources and supports? *(What is getting in the way now, and potentially in the future?)*

_____

_____

_____

_____

How can you begin working on this, what skills can you use, and what is the timeline? *(Commit to your plan)*

_____

_____

_____

_____

References

American Academy of Pain Medicine. (2015). AAPM facts and figures on pain. Retrieved from: http://www.painmed.org/PatientCenter/Facts_on_Pain.aspx (last accessed October 31, 2016).

American Cancer Society. (2013). Cancer facts & figures 2013. Retrieved from: http://www.cancer.org/acs/groups/content/@epidemiologysurveilance/documents/document/acspc-036845.pdf (last accessed October 31, 2016).

American Cancer Society. (2014). Cancer treatment and survivorship facts & figures 2014–2015. Retrieved from: http://www.cancer.org/acs/groups/content/@research/documents/document/acspc-042801.pdf (last accessed October 31, 2016).

American Childhood Cancer Organization. (2013). *Childhood cancer statistics 2012*. Kensington: American Childhood Cancer Organization.

American College of Preventative Medicine. (2015). Medication adherence – improving health outcomes. Retrieved from: http://www.acpm.org/?MedAdhereTTProviders (last accessed October 31, 2016).

American Psychiatric Association. (2013). *Diagnostic and statistical manual of mental disorders*, 5 edn. (*DSM-V*). Washington, DC: APA.

American Psychological Association (2015). Evidence-Based Practice in Psychology. Retrieved from: http://www.apa.org/practice/resources/evidence/ (last accessed October 31, 2016).

American Society of Anesthesiologists (2010). Practice guideline for chronic pain management. *Anesthesiology, 112*(4): 1–24.

Arkowitz, H. (1992). A common factors therapy for depression. In: J. C. Norcross & M. R. Goldfried (eds.), *Handbook of psychotherapy integration*. New York: Basic Books, pp. 402–432.

Baile, W. F., Buckman, R., Lenzia, R., Glober, G., Beale, E. A., & Kudelka, A. P. (2000). SPIKES – a six-step protocol for delivering bad news: Application to the patient with cancer. *The Oncologist, 5*(4): 302–311.

Baumeister, R. F. & Heatherton, T. F. (1996). Self-regulation failure: An overview. *Psychological Inquiry, 7*: 1–15.

Berg, J., Evangelista, L. S., & Dunbar-Jacob, J. (2002). Compliance. In: I. M. Lukin & P. Larsen (eds.), *Chronic illness: Impact and interventions*, 5 edn. Boston, MA: Jones and Bertlett, pp. 203–232.

Blevins, W. (1993). *Your family your self.* Oakland, CA: New Harbinger Publications.

Broadbent, E., Petrie, K. J., Main, J., & Weinman, J. (2006). The Brief Illness Perception Questionnaire (BIPQ). *Journal of Psychosomatic Research, 60:* 631–637.

Burrows, B. (2006). How stress works. Retrieved from: http://science.howstuffworks.com/environmental/life/human-biology/how-stress-works.htm (last accessed October 31, 2016).

Butler, A., Chapman, J., Forman, E., & Beck, A. (2006). The empirical status of cognitive-behavioral therapy: A review of meta-analyses. *Clinical Psychology Review, 26*(1): 17–31.

Cancer Institute NSW. (2015). What are the different stages of cancer. Retrieved from: https://www.cancerinstitute.org.au/understanding-cancer/what-are-the-different-stages-of-cancer (last accessed October 31, 2016).

Cancer Treatment Centers of America. (2014). Addressing sleep problems in cancer patients. Retrieved from: http://www.cancercenter.com/community/newsletter/article/addressing-sleep-problems-in-cancer-patients/ (last accessed October 31, 2016).

Carlson, M. (2014). *CBT for chronic pain and psychological well-being: A skills training manual integrating DBT, ACT, behavioral activation and motivational interviewing.* Chichester: John Wiley & Sons, Ltd.

Carver, C. S. & Scheier, M. F. (1998). *On the self-regulation of behavior.* New York: Cambridge University Press.

Centers for Disease Control and Prevention. (2003). Health-related quality of life (HRQOL). Retrieved from: http://www.cdc.gov/hrqol (last accessed October 31, 2016).

Centers for Disease Control and Prevention. (2011). Chronic disease overview. Retrieved from: http://www.cdc.gov/chronicdisease/overview/index.htm (last accessed October 31, 2016).

Chiles, J., Lambert, M., & Hatch, A. (1999). The impact of psychological interventions on medical cost offset: A meta-analytic review. *Clinical Psychology: Science and Practice, 6*(2): 204–220.

Colbert, S. (2013). *The process of emotional healing.* Raleigh, NC: Lulu.

Committee on Advancing Pain Research, Care, and Education, & Institute of Medicine. (2011). Relieving pain in America: A blueprint for transforming prevention, care, education, and research. Retrieved from: https://www.nationalacademies.org/hmd/~/media/Files/Report%20Files/2011/Relieving-Pain-in-America-A-Blueprint-for-Transforming-Prevention-Care-Education-Research/Pain%20Research%202011%20Report%20Brief.pdf (last accessed October 31, 2016).

de Figueiredo, J. M. & Frank, J. D. (1982). Subjective incompetence, the clinical hallmark of demoralization. *Comprehensive Psychiatry, 23*(4): 353–363.

Diefenbach, M. A. (2014). Illness representations. Retrieved from: http://cancercontrol.cancer.gov/brp/research/constructs/illness_representations.pdf (last accessed October 31, 2016).

Duncan, B. L. & Reese, R. J. (2012). The Partners for Change Outcome Management System (PCOMS): Revisiting the client's frame of reference. *Psychotherapy, 52,* 391–401.

Edelman, S., Bell, D., & Kidman, A. (1999). A group cognitive behaviour therapy programme with metastatic breast cancer patients. *Psycho-Oncology, 8*(4): 295–305

Fennell, P. A. (2003). *Managing chronic illness: Using the four-phase treatment approach.* Hoboken, NJ: John Wiley & Sons, Inc.

Frank, J. D. & Frank, J. B. (1991). *Persuasion and healing,* 3 edn. Baltimore, MD: Johns Hopkins University Press.

Gatchel, R. J. (2004). Comorbidity of chronic pain and mental health disorders: The biopsy-chosocial perspective. *American Psychologist, 59*(8): 795–805.

Gatchel, R. J., Peng, Y. B., Peters, M. L., Fuchs, P. N., & Turk, D. C. (2007). The biopsy-chosocial approach to chronic pain: Scientific advances and future directions. *Psychological Bulletin, 133*(4): 581–624.

Gilder, R., Buchsman, P., Sitartz, A., & Wolff, J. (1978). Group therapy with parents of leukaemic children. *American Journal of Psychotherapy, 32*: 276–287.

Goold, S. D. & Lipkin, M. (1999). The doctor–patient relationship. *Journal of General Internal Medicine, 14*(Suppl. 1): S26–S33.

Gottman, J. M. & Levenson, R. W. (1992). Marital processes predictive of later dissolution: Behavior, physiology, and health. *Journal of Personality and Social Psychology, 63*: 221–233.

Han, S. W., Kim, T. Y., Hwang, P. G., Jeong, S., Kim, J., Choi, I. S., et al. (2005). Predictive and prognostic impact of epidermal growth factor receptor mutation in non-small-cell lung cancer patients treated with gefitinib. *Journal of Clinical Oncology, 23*: 2493–2501.

Hayes, S. C. (1998). Thirteen rules of success: A message for students. *The Behavior Therapist, 21*, 47.

Heffner, C. (2014). Major depressive disorder (unipolar depression). Retrieved from: http://allpsych.com/disorders/mood/majordepression/ (last accessed October 31, 2016).

Kendal, W. S. & Kendal, W. M. (2012). Comparative risk factors for accidental and suicidal death in cancer patients. *Crisis, 33*(6): 325–334.

Kerns, R. D., Rosenberg, R., Jamison, R. N., Caudill, M. A., & Haythornthwaite, J. (1997). Readiness to adopt a self-management approach to chronic pain: The pain stages of change questionnaire (PSOCQ). *Pain, 72*: 227–234.

Kissane D. W., Clarke, D. M., & Street, A. F. (2001). Demoralization syndrome – a relevant psychiatric diagnosis for palliative care. *Journal of Palliative Care, 17*(1): 12–21.

Koopman, C., Butler, L., Classen, C., Giese-Davis, J., Morrow, G., Westdorf, J., et al. (2002). Traumatic stress symptoms among women with recently diagnosed primary breast cancer. *Journal of Traumatic Stress, 15*(4): 277–287.

Kübler-Ross, E. (1969). *On death and dying*. New York: The Macmillan Company.

Lau, R. R. & Hartman, K. A. (1983). Common sense representations of common illnesses. *Health Psychology, 2*, 185–197.

Lazarus, R. S. & Folkman, S. (1984). *Stress, Appraisal and Coping*. New York: Springer

Leventhal, H., Diefenbach, M. A., & Leventhal, E. A. (1992). Illness cognition: Using common sense to understand treatment adherence and affect cognition interactions. *Cognitive Therapy and Research, 16*(2): 143–163.

Lewandowski, M.J. (2006). *The chronic pain care workbook: A self-treatment approach to pain relief using the behavioral assessment of pain questionnaire*. Oakland, CA: New Harbinger Publications, Inc.

Linehan, M. M. (1993). *Skills training manual for treating borderline personality disorder*. New York: Guilford.

Linehan, M. M. (1997). Validation and psychotherapy. In: A. Bohart & L. Greenberg (eds.), *Empathy reconsidered: New directions in psychotherapy*. Washington, DC: American Psychological Association, pp. 353–392.

Linehan, M. M. (2014). *DBT skills training handouts and worksheets*, 2 edn. New York: Guilford.

Linton, S. J. & Nordin, E. (2006). A five-year follow-up evaluation of the health and economic consequences of an early cognitive-behavioral intervention for back pain: A randomized, controlled trial. *Spine, 31*: 853–858.

LiveStrong Foundation. (2015). Cancer stigma & silence around the world: A Livestrong report. Retrieved from: https://d1un1nybq8gi3x.cloudfront.net/sites/default/files/what-we-do/reports/LSGlobalResearchReport.pdf (last accessed October 31, 2016).

Miller, S. & Bergmann, S. (2012). The Outcome Rating Scale (ORS) and the Session Rating Scale (SRS). Retrieved from: http://www.slideshare.net/scottdmiller/the-ors-and-the-srs-integrating-science-and-practice-2012 (last accessed October 31, 2016).

Mischel, W., Cantor, N., & Feldman, S. (1996). Principles of self-regulation: The nature of willpower and self-control. In: E. T. Higgins & A. W. Kruglanski (eds.), *Social psychology: Handbook of principles*. New York: Guilford, pp. 329–360.

Mitchell, S., Brian, J., Zwaigenbaum, L., Roberts, W., Szatmari, P., Smith, I., et al. (2006). Early language and communication development of infants later diagnosed with autism spectrum disorder. *Developmental and Behavioral Pediatrics, 27*: S69–S78.

Monga, S., Young, A., & Owens, M. (2009). Evaluating a cognitive behavioural group program for five to seven year old children: A pilot study. *Depression and Anxiety, 27*: 243–250.

Morely, S., Eccleston, C., & Williams, A. (1999). Systemic review and meta-analysis of randomized controlled trials of cognitive behavior therapy and behavior therapy for chronic pain in adults, excluding headache. *Pain, 80*: 1–13.

Moss-Morris, R., Weinman, J., Petrie, K. J., Horne, R., Cameron, L. D., & Buick, D. (2002). The Revised Illness Perception Questionnaire (IPQ-R). *Psychology and Health, 17*: 1–16.

Multi-Health Systems. (2012). QLQ™: Quality of Life Questionnaire. Retrieved from: http://www.mhs.com/product.aspx?gr=cli&prod=qlq&id=overview (last accessed October 31, 2016).

National Cancer Institute. (2010). The future of cancer research: Accelerating scientific innovation: President's Cancer Panel annual report 2010–2011. Retrieved from: http://deainfo.nci.nih.gov/advisory/pcp/annualReports/pcp10-11rpt/FullReport.pdf (last accessed October 31, 2016).

National Cancer Institute. (2013). Psychological stress and cancer. Retrieved from: http://www.cancer.gov/about-cancer/coping/feelings/stress-fact-sheet (last accessed October 31, 2016).

National Cancer Institute. (2014). Annual report to the nation on the status of cancer, 1975–2012. Retrieved from: https://www.cancer.gov/research/progress/annual-report-nation (last accessed October 31, 2016).

National Cancer Institute (2015a). About cancer. Retrieved from: http://www.cancer.gov/about-cancer (last accessed October 31, 2016).

National Cancer Institute (2015b). A new normal. Retrieved from: http://www.cancer.gov/about-cancer/coping/survivorship/new-normal/ (last accessed October 31, 2016).

Novaco, R. W. (1983). Stress inoculation therapy for anger control. In: P. A. Keller & L. G. Ritt (eds.), *Innovations in clinical practice: A sourcebook*, Vol. 2. Sarasota, FL: Professional Resource Exchange.

Novaco, R. W. (1985). Anger control therapy. In: A. Bellack & M. Hersen (eds.), *Dictionary of behavior therapy techniques*. New York: Pergamon Press, pp. 1–4.

Ownsworth, T. (2009). A biopsychosocial perspective on adjustment and quality of life following brain tumor: A systematic evaluation of the literature. *Disability & Rehabilitation, 31*(13): 1038–1055.

Pao, M. & Weiner, L. (2011). Anxiety and depression. In: J. Wolf, P. Hinds, & B. Sourkes (eds.), *Textbook of interdisciplinary pediatric palliative care*. Philadelphia, PA: Elsevier, pp. 952–968.

Pearson. (1994). Symptom Checklist-90-Revised (SCL-90-R®). Retrieved from: http://www. pearsonclinical.com/psychology/products/100000645/symptom-checklist-90-revised-scl-90-r.html?origsearchtext=SCL-90-R (last accessed October 31, 2016).

Pederson, L. & Pederson, C. S. (2012). *The expanded dialectical behavior therapy skills training manual.* Eau Claire, WI: Premier Publishing & Media.

Pirl, W., Beck, B. J., Safren, S., & Kim, H. (2001). A descriptive study of psychiatric consultation in a community primary care center. *Primary Care Companion to the Journal of Clinical Psychiatry, 3*(5): 190–194.

Rollnick, S., Miller, W. R., & Butler, C. (2008). *Motivational interviewing in health care: Helping patients change behavior.* New York: Guilford.

Rotter, J. B. (1954). Orientation to change. In: *Social learning and clinical psychology.* New York: Prentice-Hall.

Sikora, K. (2004). Is psychosocial care worth the money? *Psycho-Oncology, 13*(12): 855–856.

Sperry, L. (2006). *Psychological treatment of chronic illness: The biopsychosocial therapy approach.* Washington, DC: APA Books.

Sperry, L. (2014). *Behavioral health: Integrating individual and family interventions in the treatment of medical conditions.* New York: Routledge.

Strang, P., Strang, S., Hultborn, R., & Arner, S. (2004). Existential pain – an entity, a provocation, or a challenge? *Journal of Pain and Symptom Management, 27*(3), 241–250.

Turk, D. C., & Flor, H. (2006). The cognitive-behavioral approach to pain management. In: S. B. McMaho & M. Koltzenberg (eds.), *Wall and Melzack's textbook of pain*, 5 edn. London: Elsevier Churchill Livingstone.

Union for International Cancer Control. (2014). 2013 annual report. Retrieved from: http://www.uicc.org/2013-annual-report (last accessed October 31, 2016).

Wampold, B. E. (2001). *The great psychotherapy debate: Models, methods, and findings.* Mahwah, NJ: Lawrence Erlbaum Associates.

Weinman, J., Petrie, K., Moss-Morris, R., & Horne, R. (1996). The Illness Perception Questionnaire: A new method for assessing the cognitive representation of illness. *Psychology and Health, 11*: 431–445.

World Health Organization. (1948). International Health Conference, New York.

Index

CBT for Psychological Well-Being in Cancer: A Skills Training Manual Integrating DBT, ACT, Behavioral Activation and Motivational Interviewing, First Edition. Mark Carlson.
© 2017 John Wiley & Sons, Ltd. Published 2017 by John Wiley & Sons, Ltd.

Printed and bound by CPI Group (UK) Ltd, Croydon, CR0 4YY

09/10/2024

14571436-0002

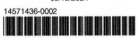